Marjorie L. Thilber

THE TRUTH ABOUT
ARTHRITIS CARE

The Truth About Arthritis Care

by

JOHN J. CALABRO, M.D.

and

JOHN WYKERT

DAVID McKAY COMPANY, INC. NEW YORK

THE TRUTH ABOUT ARTHRITIS CARE

Second Printing, October 1971

LIBRARY OF CONGRESS CATALOG CARD NUMBER: 79-161671

MANUFACTURED IN THE UNITED STATES OF AMERICA

*To our dear mothers and a
very special mother-in-law*

Contents

Preface

THIS BOOK was conceived at two bedsides 3,000 miles apart. The first was in New York, in the back wards of a chronic disease hospital, where a 29-year-old arthritis victim was ready to give up his 15-year-long fight against his disease. The other was in Los Angeles, in a great modern medical center, where a 13-year-old girl died, not from her affliction but from the effects of improper treatment.

That this could happen is one of the many shocking things about arthritis. But let me explain why these two tragic events convinced me that you—the millions of Americans who have some form of arthritis—were in need of the best, most up-to-date information about your disease.

Some years ago, while John Wykert was the science writer at the Arthritis Foundation, he received a call from a 29-year-old man who had spent half his life fighting rheumatoid arthritis. He had read in a New York paper about a new "cure" that he hoped might help him.

Unfortunately, although widely reported, this was a treatment approach that was old and long discarded as ineffective. So discouraged was the young man when he heard this that he poured out the anguish of his 15-year struggle to rout the disease that had left him crippled and unable to work, a charity patient in the back ward of a chronic disease hospital.

The recital of what the young man had endured—including the two operations he had undergone and the experimental drugs that had been tried on him—was a cry for help that John felt could not be ignored.

Consequently, he asked me to visit the young man. After examining him, it was my opinion that the young man could be helped. I felt that if he had received proper treatment from the beginning he would not have been in such poor condition or in such a hopeless frame of mind. As it turned out, the young man found a surgeon interested in his problem. When I last heard from him he was doing better, and had been weaned away from the drugs whose side effects were as severe as his disease. All I had been able to do was to provide a little encouragement.

Two years later, when John visited me, he was invited to attend the medical rounds at a renowned medical center in California. One of the patients visited that morning was a pale and sickly 13-year-old girl. Famous teachers and their students gathered around the child's bed and she sweetly and patiently answered all questions put to her.

Later, in the hall, one of the residents read aloud the girl's medical history. It was a shocking tale of years of mistreatment and misdiagnosis—some of it right in the medical center. Leaving the child and her distraught mother, the doctors withdrew into a conference room where a heated debate began about what to do next.

It was amazing that much of the discussion centered on how to counteract the previous improper care. Some of the suggested treatment was, I am afraid, little better than what had already been done for the child. Even more shocking was the sharp disagreement among the experts about what should have been done in the past and what might be done in the future.

All discussion ceased when someone entered the room with the news that the little girl had just died, not from juvenile rheumatoid arthritis, but from a deadly side effect of the drug treatment she had received.

I cannot forget this little girl's tragic fate or the outrageous fact that just a little knowledge could have saved her. For this child was on a drug that never should have been administered in the first place. This simple fact haunts me. Why didn't her doctors or her parents know this basic truth about the child's disease?

This book is my answer to all the questions the parents of this little girl were probably asking. It is directed to all arthritis patients who do not know what to do about their disease or whether they are receiving the care they need. The book is written to arm you with the truth about arthritis in order to help you make several decisions: Are you receiving the kind of treatment best suited to a specific form of arthritis? What can you expect from your disease? From your doctor's treatment? Are you doing everything you can to support your doctor's care? Here you will learn whether you should consult a specialist, or whether it may be advisable to change doctors. This book's purpose is to help all arthritis patients. But should it prevent the hopelessness or the crippling of only a single man, woman, or child, its publication will be well justified.

The premise for the book is very simple. I have never

met an arthritis patient I could not help, no matter how
severe or far advanced the arthritis may be. Yet the great
majority of arthritis patients appear to receive either little
or no help. For me this partial or inadequate care is the
most shocking truth about arthritis care today. Why
should this be happening to you?

I suspect that you, like most arthritis patients today,
are living in the past, when little could be done for arthritis. Somehow you still cling to the old "nothing can be
done" fallacy, even though the outlook for all forms of
arthritis is constantly improving. Somehow the persistent
efforts of the Arthritis Foundation, the National Institute
of Arthritis and Metabolic Diseases, or the now defunct
Diabetes and Arthritis Control Program of the National
Center for Chronic Disease Control have not as yet
reached enough people with their message of hope.

Year after year, you who have arthritis suffer in silence,
too often grasping at any remedy or cure, however unor-
thodox it may be. Frequently you either avoid doctors or
are not helped by them. Too often you may be right in
not trusting treatment. But if all arthritis patients were
more informed, doctors would have to follow suit, and
stay ahead of their patients! And this would help build up
the concern of private and public agencies, industry, and
the Government and help them to tackle the crisis in arthritis care today.

Arthritis sufferers need to become a pressure group, as
knowing about their disease as members of a trade union
are about their craft. This book hopes to provide you with
the know-how, the basic truths you need to know to gird
for the battle.

John J. Calabro
Worcester, 1971

THE TRUTH ABOUT
ARTHRITIS CARE

I. My Most Memorable Patients

> I have recently been listing the various inflammatory and degenerative conditions of joints and they number 164 to date. The layman who refers lightly to "rheumatism and arthritis," as though it were a single entity, little knows how many pathological processes can be present.
>
> F. DUDLEY HART, M.D.

MEDICAL SCHOOLS should give courses in human nature. Since they don't, it is from patients that doctors learn to be as aware of human needs as of medical problems. I am grateful, therefore, to my first and in many ways most memorable patients. They taught me about the personal dilemmas arthritis patients must overcome before I could provide effective medical care.

Far too many arthritis patients feel constantly threatened by pain, fear, and the haunting specter of becoming crippled and helpless. They are beset by self-defeating bewilderment, not knowing whom to believe, what to do, or where to turn. These confusing circumstances hamper or prevent many patients from benefiting from a realistic treatment program. Therefore, the first duty of a doctor is to educate his patient. Together they must be prepared for what lies ahead.

Surprisingly, this is the hardest task for both patients and doctors. If patients don't learn about their disease,

1

what are the alternatives? They fill the gap with eccentric treatment substitutes born of their fear and hopelessness. It is no coincidence that millions of American arthritis victims are cheated every year by a horde of "get-well-quick" quacks.

I came to rheumatology, the medical specialty of treating arthritis and rheumatism, eager to provide the ideal care I had studied so long to learn. Before I set up my first arthritis clinic in 1958, I had spent seven years in preparation, at Georgetown University Hospital, on the Harvard medical service of the Boston City Hospital, at the Massachusetts General Hospital, at the Jersey City Medical Center, and in England, at Hammersmith Hospital, London, and the Juvenile Rheumatism Unit, Taplow.

I already knew that good training is not enough. A series of disappointments was to show me that I needed to know more about the human beings in my care before I could be of help to them. From my first failures—my most memorable patients—I gained insight and understanding. Because these experiences led to subsequent successes, I want to share them with you.

THE CASE OF THE GIN AND GARLIC REMEDY

Among my first patients was Mrs. Emily Rosario, as I will call her. Her arthritis was not severe. By following a simple treatment regimen and easy home care she was sure to do well. As yet, she had only minor swellings of her hands and knees. With proper care, nothing was likely to prevent her from continuing the housework that was the most important part of her life. From the start I knew what a great cook she was, since she always brought some freshly made, tempting tid-bit that the clinic staff and I just had to taste.

Mrs. Rosario was most ingratiating. Short and round, with snow-white hair, she was friendly and enthusiastic. She endeared herself by telling me how delighted her neighborhood friends were that the Jersey City Medical Center had opened an arthritis clinic. She was also so happy that I was there—all her life she had wanted to be treated by a "nice young Italian doctor." It was a pleasant way to establish a good doctor-patient relationship, I thought.

But Mrs. Rosario's condition did not improve.

Not until much later, and after a survey done by a public health specialist, did the cause of her problem emerge. Mrs. Rosario's sister-in-law had long ago convinced Mrs. Rosario that nothing could be expected from treatment.

"You are wasting your time and money," the sister-in-law, who also had arthritis, kept telling my patient. "Those doctors know nothing. Face it, Emily, when you have arthritis, no one can prevent pain and suffering."

My efforts could not compete with these deeply ingrained views. Mrs. Rosario kept coming to me for attention and for sympathy. But advice she accepted only from her sister-in-law, and for a remedy she trusted a home brew of gin and garlic.

Mrs. Rosario was among the first of several memorable patients who presented me with this curious paradox: she had come to me, or really to the team at the arthritis clinic, to ask for help. Yet at the same time, she was sabotaging our efforts. Such resistance is not unusual, but at the time I had very little experience in coping with such behavior.

A psychiatrist once explained to me that it did not matter to him how many insights a patient achieved in his office. What he cared about was the work a patient did on his own away from the doctor, how the patient applied newly gained insights to an unhappy way of life. It is the same for arthritis patients. An arthritis patient can only be led to treatment; the doctor cannot force the patient to achieve results. After all, what are the minutes or hours a patient spends in a doctor's office compared to a lifetime of arthritis?

The burden is on the patient to help himself. Almost invariably, arthritis requires home treatment that is prescribed and supervised by a doctor, but must be carried out by the patient. This is the key concept of ideal arthritis care. I have never seen an arthritis patient I could not help in some manner. Mind you, patients who seek early treatment will fare better than those who delay. There is no cure, but no matter how long the disease has lasted or how severe it has become, something can be done to help. Effective preventive and restorative treatment has been available for arthritis patients for decades now.

But many patients expect too much too soon. They cherish the misconception that a doctor will do something mysterious *to* or *for* them that will solve their problems. In ideal arthritis care, a doctor does something quite simple *with* a patient. He helps the patient get started—with a correct diagnosis, with drugs, with an individualized home treatment regimen. The doctor then helps to keep the patient going, changing the treatment when necessary. Good results depend on what a patient does by himself. Having been properly motivated to begin treatment, patients also need to become as well-informed about their disease as they would be about other areas in their life, business, hobbies, or investments. There is no substitute for really knowing the facts. It is my theory that the more knowledgeable and sophisticated a patient is about his disease and treatment, the more he will achieve in coping with his affliction. In ideal arthritis care, the patient is an active participant, not a passive, submissive object of treatment.

I failed to motivate Mrs. Rosario to get started. As a consequence, her condition deteriorated. Her confusion—leading her to seek help and then reject it—is understandably human. There are a welter of cultural, social, economic, and psychological pressures that may defeat patients like Mrs. Rosario long before they seek treatment.

The Arthritis Foundation has compiled a list of very diverse factors that deter ideal arthritis care in our society. The arthritis victim can get short-circuited by:

A well-meaning relative or friend who says "don't waste your time with doctors because they don't know anything to do for arthritis;" and who recommends a pet home remedy.

A doctor who, unaware of what can be done, says to the patient, "There isn't much I can do for you," and fails to send the patient to a specialist or clinic where team care is available.

A medical school that minimizes arthritis training for students.

A hospital that is still geared to provide care only for acute illness and fails to adapt its services to help patients with chronic disease.

An arthritis "remedy" advertiser who lures the arthritis sufferer to try bootleg medicines or special treatment devices—expensive and worthless, thus delaying proper treatment that *can* prevent disability.

A Congressman on a health appropriations committee who gives low priority to funds for arthritis research and training, but high priority to funding research against the glamorous "killer" diseases (the National Institute of Arthritis and Metabolic Diseases's 1968 budget was $137,281,000 with less than 15 percent of that amount channeled for arthritis).

A Government health official who says drugs for chronic diseases should be covered under Medicare, except those for arthritis because it would be too costly.

An advertiser of aspirin who, in promoting a legitimate and useful product, encourages the patient to treat himself, when the proper aspirin dosage should *always* be prescribed by a qualified physician for each individual patient.

A book publisher who uses sensational advertising to promote a volume containing nonsense about overcoming or "curing" arthritis with health foods or enemas or mud baths or self-hypnotism, et cetera ad nauseam.

A chiropractor who is not a medical doctor, who is incorrect in his idea of what causes arthritis symptoms, and who in his spinal and other manipulations can do serious damage.

An employer who, fearful of absenteeism, declines to hire the arthritic.

An insurance company that penalizes the arthritis sufferer by charging higher rates for health insurance.

A broadcaster who gives air time and free publicity to promoters of fraudulent, misrepresented, or merely misguided "remedies" for arthritis.

A newspaper that accepts questionable arthritis advertising without first checking the Better Business Bureau, the Arthritis Foundation, or some watchdog agency.

The arthritis victim himself who, instead of organizing with other arthritics to demand action to combat their mutual problem, seems apathetically to accept his fate.

THE CASE OF THE MAN WHO
LIED TO HIMSELF

Obvious or subtle, these forces cause misunderstanding, despair, and gullibility. And don't for a minute believe that it is only the Mrs. Rosarios of this world who succumb. For as the famous Dr. William Osler observed, "In all matters relating to disease, credulity remains a permanent fact, uninfluenced by civilization or education."

How else can one explain Frank Farrell?

Frank was having backaches severe enough to wake him. In the morning, after he had moved around a little, he found that the backache disappeared. After several months of recurrent discomfort, Frank discovered that by stooping a little he was able to ease his pain. This he continued to do for some time. He assumed that the backache was caused by tension or the weight he had gained since leaving college, so he determined to go to his athletic club more often, and to exercise rather than just settle for his usual massage.

But his pain grew worse. He was stooping almost all the time. A doctor he consulted told him it was a case of too much tension and that he should lose weight and exercise. When he finally came to see me, he had been suffering for close to a year from a life-long arthritic condition known as ankylosing spondylitis.

Frank's competitive drives were all-consuming. Born poor, he was determined to be rich. In high school, he played basketball with the same drive he was later to show in business. He won an athletic scholarship to a prestigious Ivy-League school where he did as well in his studies as on the basketball court. After graduation, he joined a major corporation where he was now a senior vice president. He had reached the top at only 37.

Now he was on an endless round of business trips, going to luncheons, dinner meetings, and social functions that were part of his increased business responsibilities. In private life he felt unchanged, a deprived poor boy hungering for success. Tall, handsome, and looking much younger than his years, Frank was troubled. But he promised himself that he would soon let up on the frantic pace and enjoy life with his wife.

Despite his crowded schedule, Frank was always punctual for his appointments, and never failed to show up, although he was out of town most of the time. But he also failed to show any improvement.

Unlike Mrs. Rosario, Frank Farrell did not consciously "resist" treatment. He listened to what I said, and seemed to understand. He took his medication, and he spent all the time he was supposed to with the clinic's physiatrist —the doctor who specializes in physical medicine and, in Frank's case, the professional who taught the exercises Frank was to do each day. These were quite different from the ones he had performed to ease his backache— which had actually promoted his stooping over, instead of preventing the gradual deformity. What, then, was the matter?

I had assumed that Frank, an aggressive, successful executive, would attack his own problem of arthritis the way he would solve a business dilemma—that he would try to find out what the problem was all about, seek a solution, and, having found one, carry it out. But that is where I made my mistake. Unlike Mrs. Rosario, who resisted treatment, Frank Farrell denied the fact that his illness was serious and that he would have to combat it for life. This denial influenced the measures he took to prevent his condition from getting worse. Taking the drug I prescribed was only the first step. He had also been instructed to spend three half-hour periods each day doing a set of simple exercises to help prevent his stoop from developing into a poker back. These exercises could be done at home or in the office, or in a hotel room during a trip. His failure to exercise was not because this was difficult or inconvenient. Having denied the existence and nature of his illness, he also ignored the importance of doing therapeutic exercises.

Because of his excellent self-control, I was unaware of Frank's emotional problems. Outwardly he was pleasant and appeared to be cooperative. Inwardly insecure, he felt unsafe on the top of his success ladder—one step and he would surely fall. The step that could cause this catastrophe was to admit he had a chronic, crippling disease.

It was not my intuition that helped me to discover Mrs. Rosario's resistance and Mr. Farrell's denial. Small bits of evidence are gathered by everyone at the clinic—including our secretary, the nurses, the social worker, and the medical specialists who make up the arthritis treatment team, the biochemist who heads the laboratory, the technicians, the other doctors on the staff, and the consultants, such as the surgeon, the psychiatrist, the podiatrist who examines the patients' feet or the ophthalmologist who examines their eyes.

What are these bits of evidence? The idle, seemingly meaningless, remarks made by patients. Often, they reveal the emotional turmoil that is part of the initial reaction to arthritis.

WHAT YOU REVEAL ABOUT YOURSELF

The importance of what patients say has been pointed out by two investigators in the psychiatry department of Stanford University School of Medicine. Working with a small group of women with rheumatoid arthritis, George F. Solomon, M.D., and Rudolf H. Moos, Ph.D., compiled a list of phrases taken from a psychological test that in their experiments helped to differentiate the patients who were likely to respond well to treatment from those who were not.

Those who would not do well would say things like:
- I have not lived the right kind of life.
- No one seems to understand me.
- My hardest battles are with myself.
- I wish I were not so shy.
- It makes me uncomfortable to put on a stunt at a party even when others are doing the same sort of thing.
- My sleep is fitful and disturbed.
- I have a great deal of stomach trouble.
- Whenever possible I avoid being in a crowd.
- I feel like giving up quickly when things go wrong.
- I find it hard to keep my mind on a task or job.
- I brood a great deal.
- Criticism or scolding hurts me terribly.
- I have had very peculiar and strange experiences.
- I have often felt that strangers were looking at me critically.
- I am easily embarrassed.
- I am easily downed in an argument.

By contrast, patients who were likely to respond well to treatment would say:

- I have very few quarrels with members of my family.
- I do not tire quickly.
- I have very few headaches.
- My sex life is satisfactory.
- My daily life is full of things that keep me interested.
- I believe that my home life is as pleasant as that of most people I know.
- I seem to be about as capable and smart as most others around me.
- I have no dread of going into a room by myself where other people have already gathered and are talking.
- I do not mind being made fun of.
- I enjoy the excitement of a crowd.
- I seem to make friends about as quickly as others do.

By comparing the two lists of phrases, it is immediately apparent that patients who are happy with themselves and the lives they lead will also be the good and satisfied patients. Obviously, I could not improve the lives of the patients who saw me. But trying to provide proper treatment in the face of patients' negative attitudes made for unexpected troubles.

For instance, I had failed to help a 16-year-old fledgling ballerina. Sonia was stricken with rheumatoid arthritis that affected her left knee. She saw her life in ruins, her planned career a hopeless dream. Her mother, who seemed to be living through her only child, was even more grief-stricken. Although I explained repeatedly that chances were excellent that Sonia would walk normally and, possibly, even dance again, the emotional crisis brought on by the illness outweighed my reasoning. They were mourning a career that had yet to materialize, instead of marshaling their resources to cope with the problem at hand. After a few visits, Sonia stopped treatment, and to this day I do not know what happened.

Another vain attempt was to help Walter, a lawyer who developed gout while in his early 30s. An irrational, ill-tempered man, he had to be practically blackmailed by his wife before he would come to the clinic. At his age he felt he could not possibly have an arthritic condition. Despite his educational level, he simply refused to believe that untreated gout could cripple. He was unreachable and consequently untreatable.

George, a 50-ish cocktail-lounge pianist, had to stop working because rheumatoid arthritis had begun to twist his fingers. He refused to consider a series of small operations that would have restored almost normal function to his hands. He agreed that the operation would be helpful, but was afraid that he would die from the anesthesia the way his father had many years ago. Somehow we finally got him to go to the hospital. But then he refused to sign the permission to operate. His fingers became so twisted that he could not hold a pencil or button his jacket. Although an operation might still help, he continues to refuse the surgery.

Most upsetting was Rachel Warner, the innocent victim of her parents' deluded desperation. Rachel, a beautiful five-year-old, had juvenile rheumatoid arthritis. By the time I examined her, she had been seriously ill for many months. Her parents had rushed her from doctor to doctor before I correctly diagnosed her disease. The parents assumed that I would now bring about a speedy "cure."

Almost at once I found that the Warners provided almost none of the essential home care that Rachel required. Mrs. Warner had also trained Rachel never to tell what was done at home so that I could not scold or criticize. Before I could take the parents to task, they disappeared altogether.

Two years later, they brought Rachel back to me. I was appalled. Rachel was suffering from the after-effects of a so-called new "wonder drug," available only from a doctor in Montreal. The drug is a dangerous combination of cortisone and male and female hormones. Although Rachel was only seven years old, the drug had caused her to menstruate, to grow pubic hair, and to develop a fungus infection of the nails on her hands and feet. And even these problems were minor compared to the condition of her hips.

The relatively large doses of cortisone were perhaps responsible for the fact that Rachel's hips had begun to disintegrate. This in turn caused a curvature of the spine; she looked crippled and was barely able to move. It was hard to say whether the disease or the medication had caused the harm done.

Even then, something could be done for her. But it took a long time before most of the damage could be repaired. Surgery reversed the hip problem. Rachel now walks with only a little difficulty. She attends a regular school and participates in most activities. Instead of a miracle drug, Rachel faithfully takes her prescribed aspirin. Her disease is under good control, particularly since her parents work on her exercises with her. This regimen should have been followed from the start. Rachel's disastrous difficulties were unnecessary, the result of the Warners' unreasonable expectations of "instant cure" and the greed of a disreputable Canadian doctor. Fortunately, the parents have come to terms with Rachel's chronic disease. Cooperation and understanding have taken the place of their former "fight and flight" relationship with doctors.

These difficult patients and their problems were becoming of increasing concern to me and to the other staff members of the arthritis clinic. In many staff conferences we tried to determine what it was that troubled our patients. We agreed that arthritis had an unexpectedly devastating impact on a disproportionately large number of victims. What was it, this state of siege caused by the affliction?

It was the impression of the clinic staff that patients fretted about their age—they thought they were stigmatized by an "old-age" disease. Whatever their age, the image they had of themselves as being young was shattered. Suddenly, we concluded, they felt excluded from our youth-oriented culture.

Guilt obsessed many patients. Although patients were repeatedly told that no one knows the cause of various forms of arthritis, nonetheless, they constantly asked themselves where they had gone wrong. Was it an improper diet, exposure to inclement weather, the development of bad work or rest habits? No answer about the cause of their disease seemed to ease these doubts.

The specter of crippling haunted almost every patient, even those most unlikely to suffer any disability. Their reaction really depended on how they had viewed afflicted people before they themselves became ill. If they viewed "cripples" with horror or disdain, their own reaction to relatively mild symptoms of pain, stiffness, or restricted movement was intense.

A combination of these tumultuous emotions very often resulted in a form of "contained hatred." Patients loathed themselves and tried to conceal it. Their hatred of the clinic and its staff similarly smoldered. Only a few patients, it seemed to us, were able to show their anger openly. Some walked out on us. Parents of children with rheumatoid arthritis often had the same set of reactions that the patients themselves displayed. If angry, they would yank their children out of the clinic.

Most patients, though, felt very ambivalent. For example, Mrs. Rosario and Frank Farrell punished us by not doing well, although she brought us food and claimed to love us, while he was always punctual and made a great show of good-humored cooperation.

The varied and complex emotions engendered by arthritis surprised me, but they should not have. After all, my determination to succeed as an arthritis specialist had its own emotional roots. I was in high school when my mother became incapacitated from rheumatoid arthritis. Her four sisters already had the same disease. At the time, it seemed to me that I was part of a doomed family. It was not until later that I was to realize that such familial illness is not particularly rare. We had not been singled out to suffer. But suffer we did.

Seething with resentment, but giving a brave show of courage, my two brothers and I took over the household chores our mother was incapable of doing. I seem always to have ended up with a task I despised. It must have been over one of those bubbling pots of pasta I was always stirring that I made the vow to help—I would dedicate my life to ease suffering and become an arthritis specialist.

This decision, which I have no reason to regret, was born under pressure. It emerged from highly emotional feelings and hateful circumstances.

In reflecting on this I began to realize that it was now my task to channel the self-hate and other mixed emotions of my patients into similarly affirmative action.

I had to change my approach, I realized. Because I had been principally interested in the medical, not the human, facts of arthritis, I had used scientific medicine to treat my patients. I now understood that there were other approaches that I could not ignore. Patients cling to "primitive medicine," which assumes that disease causes are magical; they also believe in "folk medicine," which resorts to the hit-or-miss application of traditional home remedies. I could not apply what I knew without also taking into account that sin, guilt, or punishment are all associated by patients with their disease state. At the same time, many patients were haunted by fears that I found irrational. Patients were afraid of disability, crippling, economic insecurity, their own low self-esteem coupled with their being downgraded as "inferior" by their family and friends.

My series of setbacks had already shown me that I needed to understand human nature, to let human nature teach me. The clinic staff and I needed to know right from the start what our patients were thinking and feeling. What did they really know about their disease *after* we had spent considerable time explaining it to them? What did we think patients knew? How did the patients feel about themselves? And the treatment they were receiving? We were prepared to strip away our illusions.

Fortunately, at the time the staff and I were struggling with these problems—to "humanize" ourselves and to become more accessible to our patients—we had unexpected good luck. Dr. Margaret H. Edwards, now of the Public Health Service, began a study of 100 of our patients and 12 doctors associated with the clinic. Her aim was to provide the answers to our questions. With the help of our social worker, Miss Marion E. Wied, she prepared 28 questions. We asked the 100 patients, 71 of whom were women, please to be absolutely frank in their answers. That was the only way we could help one another.

However, we were not ready for the shock of what we learned.

It seemed that our patients felt we paid little attention to their complaints, questions, doubts, or fears.

How else could one interpret the finding that 64 patients wanted to know more about their disease, 28 thought their physicians were not interested in their illness, 17 felt that treatment was worse than being ill?

But there was more dismay in store for us.

Most patients knew the disease they had. But 12 of the 24 patients with osteoarthritis did not. Also, 21 of 79 patients with active disease were not aware of their condition.

The mainstay of all therapy, regular home treatment, was being ignored: Only 45 of the 70 patients supposed to take heat treatments did so. Only eight of 43 patients were getting the prescribed massages. Nine patients were not doing any exercise, the most essential part of home care. Altogether, it appeared that patients under 45 tended to ignore what we had prescribed.

We were unhappy to learn how patients rated treatment. Ten felt there was no satisfactory treatment. Sixty-three thought drugs were "the best treatment," even though we had stated over and over again that drugs by themselves were inadequate in helping arthritis patients.

The image we had formed of our patients did not correspond with the one they had of themselves. For instance, there were 46 patients whom the doctors found to have some sort if impairment; only 32 admitted to any deformity. One-third of the patients interviewed felt that their disease had made them unattractive. Since the great majority of the patients surveyed were women, this opinion may have been their unique point of view. Very few of the patients who felt unattractive had any physical impairment that might conceivably prompt this feeling. The reasons they cited for feeling repellent were "an unhappy expression all the time," looking "drawn and stiff," no longer walking naturally—it took "so long to get to the bus."

Many patients confirmed our suspicion that they thought they had become ill because of some mistake they had made. They lived in the wrong place—one-third blamed the bad weather; 20 said it was a matter of nervousness. Seventeen patients blamed an accident, 14 "hard work." Not one remembered that no one knows what causes the major forms of arthritis. Our patients thought bad diets, infections, poor teeth, acid or "bad" blood, infected tonsils, overweight, or a "dropped" stomach were responsible. "Causes" were linked to unpleasant events in the patients' lives—a financial crisis, loss of a family member, illness, an operation, working in a damp environment, moving—all of them preceded the onset or the worsening of their disease.

The most amazing and upsetting finding was the extent of self-medication practiced by the patients. Among the 100 patients, there were 160 modes of treatment suggested by friends, relatives, or neighbors. They ranged from the wearing of copper bracelets to going to Arizona. Three-quarters of the patients were either receiving chiropractic treatment, or drinking herb teas, vinegar and honey, cod liver oil, or fruit juices. It was from the questionnaire that we discovered Mrs. Rosario's devotion to gin and garlic.

Other patients rubbed themselves with salves of various kinds, iodine, kerosene, and "Chinese Tiger Balm." All these treatments were of course unknown to the staff of the clinic. When the patients were asked if they had ever told their doctor about any of these medications, they replied "he never asked me."

The survey changed all of us. We made certain we knew what our patients thought and felt about their disease. From that point on we did not assume anything about our patients' knowledge or attitudes. We found out. Predictably, we had fewer "difficult" patients and, when we did, achieved better results with them.

In a report in a medical journal, Dr. Edwards had noted that "even in a special clinic staffed by physicians with a particular interest in arthritis, there are gaps between the concepts of disease and its management held by the patient and his doctor, gaps of which neither is fully aware." This, fortunately, was no longer true of our clinic.

In getting closer to our patients, the staff sometimes changed roles. For instance, whenever I had a new young patient with juvenile rheumatoid arthritis, I would meet with the parents and our social worker for an hour or two so that I could fully explain the child's disease, its course and treatment, and what the outlook and progress were likely to be. At the conclusion of what was almost a formal lecture, I would always ask if there were any questions. Most often, the parents said they understood and they had no questions.

But on several occasions when the social worker remained with the parents after I had left or had been called away, the parents asked a torrent of questions. They had been either too stunned or shocked, or too hesitant, to ask me. But they wanted to learn more and in the process expressed their fears and doubts. Such difficulty in reaching one another—in my communicating with parents—could be easily resolved. The social worker was often better equipped than I to get parents to understand and to cooperate. We both took turns in talking to the parents until they and we were satisfied that we understood each other. The staff member the patient preferred did the educating.

There was no reason that the other doctors or I had to be the only source of knowledge. As a treatment team, we were all knowledgeable; questions could be answered by everyone. In fact, we urged greater discussion of individual patient's problems at our staff conferences. All of this was the beginning of greatly increased effectiveness. Perhaps the survey was the most important factor that forged my associates and myself into a treatment team.

For instance, we had noted that Mrs. Rosario was especially close to our secretary. When we learned about Mrs. Rosario's sister-in-law and the gin and garlic, we suggested that, while chatting with Mrs. Rosario, the secretary should invite both ladies to a clinic open house.

They came and, with a lot of other patients, were taken on a complete tour of the facility; they went into the laboratory, they talked to the technicians and to other patients. Then a box lunch was served. There Mrs. Rosario and her sister-in-law had the opportunity to talk to doctors and nurses as friends. A great many concerns of all patients were discussed. Especially important was the progress the ladies could observe in other patients, some of whom they had known before their arthritis had been brought under control.

It took only a half a day, but we could tell that Mrs. Rosario was impressed. Her sister-in-law became a patient of our clinic very soon afterwards. Now that I am in New England and Dr. Joseph Marchesano heads the clinic, they still attend and are participating in their treatment, and doing very well. No one mentions gin and garlic; now the ladies drink the brew because they want to, not as a substitute for treatment.

For Frank Farrell we arranged a group education session with other ankylosing spondylitis patients. He quickly got their message—they ·also were young and successful. But unlike Frank most of them had arranged their lives so that the disease was handled properly, not ignored.

From Frank's eventual participation in the lively group discussion, I knew he was about to climb another rung on the ladder of success; he was about to fight his fears and concentrate his attack on his disease. He was demonstrating that with greater motivation and better education he could relax about his disease, for he would soon know where he was heading and why. You will learn about Frank's considerable progress in Chapter VI.

My most memorable patients taught me the most important lesson I was to learn as an arthritis specialist: It is not enough to treat a disease; one must help educate and motivate the human being with the disease.

Whenever a patient moves—reacts to the arthritis as if fighting off a murderous attacker—then I feel at ease knowing this patient will do well, no matter how severe or difficult the disease. And I have also learned that patients who are uneducated about their disease, unmotivated, and uncooperative in their treatment will often fare badly, even when their disease is mild.

Your choice is obvious. Learning about the disease you have, finding out what needs to be done and what to expect provides important truths. These truths make you free to act. And you had better act. For if you do not do something about your arthritis, the consequences may be tragic. Too many arthritis patients do not see a doctor until they are at the point of becoming crippled. The Metropolitan Life Insurance Company points out that "many older persons are needlessly stoical in the face of the discomfort of arthritis." According to the *Statistical Bulletin* of February 1967, "Many, especially those with lower incomes, may not seek medical aid for a condition which they consider among the unpleasant and inevitable consequences of growing old."

But whether old or young, rich or poor, this is too often the experience for the roughly 17 million Americans—13 million women, four million men, and thousands of children—who are afflicted with one or another form of arthritis. This means one out of every 11 people in this country is affected, and that one out of every four U.S. families in some way feels the impact of this group of diseases. In terms of suffering, arthritis probably outranks the killer diseases (such as cancer, heart or kidney disease, or stroke). Sad to say, much of this suffering could be eased by a little education. Such education is certainly everyone's basic right. And it *is* available, from chapters of the Arthritis Foundation or from the National Institute of Arthritis and Metabolic Diseases (in Bethesda, Md.). Unfortunately, far too few arthritis victims take advantage of the educational opportunities afforded them. Yet, as you read on you will find it is easy to learn about arthritis.

THE ORIGINAL MEANINGS

Even the most knowledgeable people are often surprised, even stunned, by how little they know about arthritis and rheumatism. Take "arthritis." The word is in common use, or, more precisely, misuse. Arthritis actually means the *inflammation* of a joint; yet, even the specialists use the word to describe the degeneration or destruction of joints. *Joints*, referred to frequently in any discussion of arthritis, are the points of contact between two bones of the skeleton as well as the structures that surround and support them. The knee, the elbow, the hip, the wrist, the fingers, all contain joints that move, or articulate. In arthritis, such movement is compromised by pain, stiffness, or discomfort due to swelling of the bones, muscles, tendons, ligaments, and other component structures that comprise the joint.

Many people use "arthritis" to describe aching muscles, but this is incorrect. More appropriate is the old-fashioned and now generally discarded word "rheumatism." The word derives from the Greek word *rheuma*, which means literally "to flow" as a watery discharge (as a concept, this dates back to ancient times, when physicians believed that pain of muscles and joints was due to an "evil humor" that flowed from the brain). Rheumatism describes muscle pain, or pain in the supporting structure of the joint, such as the fibrous connecting tissues, but not in the joint itself. Because it is so nonspecific, the term rheumatism is confusing and essentially meaningless, and is now in disuse, particularly among physicians. Nonetheless, today, arthritis and rheumatism are often used interchangeably, and, therefore, have lost their original meaning. In medicine, both terms have gradually been replaced by the designation "rheumatic diseases."

There is hardly a human being alive who does not suffer from a little rheumatism every now and then. Undoubtedly, the first to suffer the twinges of rheumatism were the cavemen, whose surviving bones testify to their having had arthritis also. All rheumatic diseases have been known as "arthritis" since about 500 B.C. The word "rheumatism" seems not to have come into use until almost a thousand years later, and was probably first used by Galen, the greatest doctor of medieval times. So the present confusion about the meaning of arthritis and rheumatism is centuries old. I suspect that for the past 2,500 years, mankind has suffered from soft tissue complaints that they have mistakenly labeled "arthritis."

THE RHEUMATIC DISEASES

Their great number is the most surprising aspect of the rheumatic diseases. The American Rheumatism Association, the only professional association of arthritis specialists in the United States, is still in the process of determining and categorizing about a hundred disorders that constitute "arthritis and rheumatism" under the all-embracing term of the rheumatic diseases (or arthritides, the plural of arthritis). There are 13 different categories of rheumatic diseases. But all you need to know about are *arthritis of unknown cause*—including rheumatoid arthritis, in both adult and juvenile forms, and ankylosing spondylitis; *degenerative joint disease*—osteoarthritis or osteoarthrosis; *connective tissue disorders*—systemic lupus erythematosus, scleroderma; *arthritis associated with biochemical abnormalities*, such as gout; *arthritis associated with infections; traumatic arthritis*. These various and different diseases have one feature in common—there is pain or discomfort in the joints or surrounding tissue.

THE JOINT

One cannot begin to understand the rheumatic diseases without knowing what a joint is. The joint itself is absolutely essential to man since it allows him to move; without the structure of a joint there is no grasping or lying, sitting, standing, walking, running, jumping, moving of objects, lifting, bending, waving, exercising, and so on. A joint is a structure where two bones meet, supported by muscles and tendons that permit the bone to move up, down, and sideways. In the normal joint, the end of each bone is covered by a smooth, white, elastic substance called cartilage. This dense and fibrous kind of tissue is extremely smooth and is lubricated; this allows the bone ends to move within the joint socket. Cartilage also absorbs the mechanical shock as well as the wear and tear as a joint is used.

All joints are enclosed in a baglike structure, a capsule made up of tough fibrous tissue that is attached to the ends of the bones and keeps the joint together and in place. Within the capsule around the joint there is a soft, cushionlike material that provides the all-important lubricant to keep the joint moving. This lining is called the synovium or synovial membrane. The pale yellow, heavy, viscous liquid this membrane produces is called the synovial fluid. Without this lubricating fluid, the joint is unable to move.

Each structure of the joint is important, and any change or disorder can have serious consequences; but especially vital is that nothing happens to the fluid that serves to lubricate the cartilage at the end of the bones. A good many forms of arthritis begin with some kind of infection or inflammation of the synovial fluid (or the synovial membrane) which then spreads to the cartilage, tendons, muscles, and bones of the joint. Herewith are brief descriptions of some important forms of rheumatic diseases.

ANKYLOSING SPONDYLITIS

Also known as rheumatoid spondylitis or Marie-Strümpell disease, this is a systemic disorder that primarily affects men in their late adolescent or young adult years. It begins rather insidiously with arthritis, but most often is characterized by back pain, stiffness, and loss of function resulting from involvement of spinal joints. The poker-back, hunched-over look is the ultimate fate of those who receive little or no treatment. Pain-relieving and anti-inflammatory drugs are quite effective, however. Specifically designed exercises, training in correct posture to prevent deformity, and correction of existing deformities are also a vital part of treatment. Much progress has been made in treating this disorder, as you will read in Chapter VI.

BURSITIS

A bursa is a small sac containing fluid, which is usually situated between a tendon and the bone over which the tendon glides. Bursitis, the inflammation of a bursa, is extremely common and is a self-limiting, temporary form of rheumatism. Applying heat, resting the painful area, and taking aspirin are the most usual and effective treatments. If severe, some injections of an anti-inflammatory agent directly into the site of maximum pain may be required. Copper bracelets, much loved by athletes, are decorative but of little use in either preventing or treating bursitis.

The basic problem in bursitis is inflammation and degeneration or wear and tear of connective tissue, and researchers are attempting to learn more about the disease process by gaining a greater knowledge of the chemistry and metabolism of connective tissue. The search for more effective and less toxic drugs to treat bursitis also continues.

Conditions you know as "tennis elbow," "housemaid's knee," "frozen shoulder," "wry neck" (torticollis), "policeman's heel," tendinitis (an inflamed tendon), are low-grade inflammations of tendons, bursa, or structures around the joint. Even when these conditions seem overwhelmingly painful, treatment of these benign types of disorders will be effective and leave hardly a trace of ever having existed. Only very rarely may an operation be required.

Among other relatively brief, self-limiting conditions are arthritis due to an infection—for which antibiotics are quickly effective—the various types of "painful shoulder," and the very common ailment, low-back strain.

GOUT

Of all forms of arthritis, gout can be most successfully controlled. This is because highly effective drugs have recently been developed. One important cause of this acute, very painful, and sometimes destructive and even fatal form of arthritis is an inherited metabolic disorder associated with a build-up of uric acid and its salts in the blood and tissues. This material crystallizes and accumulates in and around the joints, resulting in inflammation, severe pain, and eventual destruction of normal joint structure.

Drugs are used to rid the body of its excess uric acid via the urine, or to prevent its formation in large quantities so that no build-up of harmful crystal deposits occurs. Researchers are now seeking the basic defect that causes the uric acid build-up.

INFECTIOUS ARTHRITIS

Once upon a time, this was the type of arthritis considered when a joint became red, hot, and swollen. Now, it is hardly thought of at all. If diagnosed correctly, it is the most readily curable form of arthritis. Seen at any age and in either sex, infectious arthritis disappeared as a major problem with the advent of penicillin and the antibiotic drugs.

Infectious arthritis can be dangerous, since bacteria are capable of damaging a joint swiftly, perhaps even in a matter of 10 days. To prevent damage, treatment formerly was often surgical; the infected fluid was drained from the affected joint. When effective drugs became available, the joint fluid was often tested and an antibiotic specific for the infecting organism was then prescribed. In due time, streptococcal, tuberculous, pneumococcal, or gonococcal arthritis, once so common, became relatively rare.

However, one type, gonococcal arthritis, appears to be resurgent; a plague to adults, children, and even newborn infants. This is so because the incidence of gonococcal arthritis parallels the spread of gonorrhea. Currently, this type of VD is spreading like wildfire, with experts predicting more than two million cases a year.

Gonococcal arthritis mostly affects the larger joints, the wrists, knees, and ankles. If untreated, extensive destruction of cartilage and bone may result. Particularly disturbing is the appearance of this type of infectious arthritis among children. Some of my patients have been between the ages of 4 and 14. One recent study showed that up to

10 percent of expectant mothers seen in a public clinic have undetected gonorrhea; consequently, gonococcal arthritis in newborn infants may become more frequent. Another source of consternation is the recent finding of resistant gonorrhea strains which may complicate treatment. Whether this means the end of one-shot treatment remains to be seen.

All you need to remember is that a diagnosis of gonococcal arthritis will again be considered if only one joint is red, hot, and swollen, that this type of arthritis is eminently treatable, and that shame gets you nowhere. *Nice* people do contract gonorrhea, and there is only one reaction that makes sense. Seek proper treatment.

OSTEOARTHRITIS

Osteoarthritis is considered part of aging, but this is not necessarily so. English researchers reported that changes due to osteoarthritis begin by the age of 25, and by the time people are 65, close to two-thirds of the population may be expected to suffer pain and disability. What happens is that joint cartilage degenerates—becomes soft, wears down unevenly, or even completely, so that the bone becomes exposed or may thicken. The main difference between so-called "osteo" and rheumatoid arthritis is that in osteo the rest of the body is rarely affected. The disorder rarely causes severe deformity or crippling, except when the hip joints are involved. Typically, osteo affects the tips of the fingers of the hand, rheumatoid arthritis the middle joints of the fingers and knuckles.

Osteo almost always occurs in middle-aged and older people. It is the remarkable aspect of this form of arthritis that an older person may have extensive osteo of the spine without feeling any pain or discomfort. Like rheumatoid arthritis, osteo seems to be more prevalent in women than men. In women, the first symptoms of pain and stiffness usually occur at the time of menopause, often in the finger joints or in those that bear the body's weight. Osteo is as old as man, and in fact has been found in the skeletons of prehistoric animals. Man and beast share this affliction, perhaps the oldest chronic disease to plague this planet.

PSORIATIC ARTHRITIS

Arthritis affects a small percentage of patients with psoriasis, a fairly common skin disease. It is still not known what causes the psoriasis or the arthritis. There is some evidence that psoriasis may be hereditary, but this has not yet been proved conclusively. New and potent drugs, several still in the experimental stage, appear to hold promise as effective forms of therapy of this complicated form of arthritis.

REITER'S SYNDROME

This form of arthritis combines urethritis (inflammation of the urethra, the passage through which urine is discharged from the bladder), arthritis, and conjunctivitis (inflammation of the delicate membrane that lines the eyelids). It has been linked with venereal disease, and occurs most commonly in young male adults. Treatment includes the use of arthritis drugs and antibiotics for the urinary infection.

Strong evidence has been found by Drs. Ephraim Engleman and Julius Schachter that one causative agent in Reiter's syndrome is a Bedsonia virus. These microorganisms have been reported to cause arthritis in lambs, and they are known to cause several other diseases in man. These investigators have produced arthritis in monkeys by injecting them with Bedsonia organisms taken from human patients with Reiter's syndrome. They were then able to recover Bedsonia virus from all the infected joints and from various internal organs of the experimental monkeys. This line of research is being pursued intensively for further evidence and for more effective treatment.

RHEUMATOID ARTHRITIS

Rheumatoid arthritis is the most crippling type of arthritis. What makes it so dangerous is that it goes beyond doing damage to the joints and supportive tissues and affects body organs such as the heart. There are constitutional symptoms—patients lose weight and feel weak, even as the disease begins by causing inflammatory changes and swelling in the membranes lining one or more joints.

Because rheumatoid arthritis is a generalized disease, the physician must "treat the entire patient, not just his joints." Because numerous other conditions resemble rheumatoid arthritis, a definitive diagnosis is difficult at times, especially when a patient's disease is not "typical" or when a patient fails to respond to treatment.

Rheumatoid arthritis occurs three times more often in women than in men and usually begins in a woman's most productive, child-bearing years, between 20 and 45. However, both sexes are susceptible at all ages, from early infancy to old age.

The cause of the disease remains unknown; it is known that climate plays no distinct role in the development or course of the disease. Rheumatoid arthritis has been found in all parts of the world. Among the most interesting studies in the prevalence of the disease has been the comparison of two tribes of Indians, one living in Northern cold and wet climate, the other in the dry Southwest. No real difference in the amount of rheumatic diseases could be found. Climate, in other words, is neither a cause nor a contributing factor. For a detailed discussion see Chapter II.

SYSTEMIC LUPUS ERYTHEMATOSUS (SLE)

A rare, generalized disease of connective tissue, SLE is manifested by structural and functional changes in the skin, joints, and internal organs. It is found most often in the 20 to 40 age group, affecting women more frequently than men. Although certain measures can be taken, there is no specific and complete treatment for this disease.

In the last few years, much progress has been made toward understanding how SLE develops. There is evidence that SLE may be the result of a disorder in the body's production of antibodies.

TRAUMATIC ARTHRITIS

This is a short-lived condition that occurs when you hit a knee or an elbow. Ordinarily, there are slight swelling and pain that eventually disappear. If you have injured yourself badly enough, the traumatized joint may become so painful that a doctor may want to remove accumulated fluid in the joint. He does this primarily to relieve pressure, but he may also want to analyze the joint fluid to make certain that the pain is due to the injury, rather than to another condition such as infectious arthritis.

Traumatic arthritis clears up fairly rapidly and by itself, with the pain readily controlled by aspirin or a doctor-prescribed pain killer. If the condition persists for more than a week or ten days, you should consult a physician to make sure that you haven't torn something within the joint or perhaps sustained a small fracture of one of the bones of the joint. Resting the joint may be suggested by your doctor, or he may ask you to apply heat; I suspect also that he will ask you to be patient, to take it easy, and to allow natural healing to take its course.

For the great majority of people, this short list of rheumatic conditions may come as a source of shock and surprise.

We never knew there were so many, these people will exclaim. We had no idea that arthritis was so complex, or that there is so much known about so many forms! Such exclamations are the beginning of knowledge, and knowledge can be turned into the power of doing something for yourself, and perhaps for others as well.

II. *My Typical Patient: The Housewife with Rheumatoid Arthritis*

Educated men are as much superior to uneducated men
as the living are to the dead.

ARISTOTLE

AN ATTRACTIVE young married woman, the mother of
three children, has just walked into my office. As she sits
at my desk, she recounts her trouble. For some time now
she has been much more tired than usual, she has felt
"sore and stiff," and has been bothered by generalized
aches and pains in her joints. Gradually, both hands have
become painfully swollen, feel hot to the touch, and are
exquisitely tender. Because she has no appetite, she has
been losing weight. She feels weak in a way she never did
before. She is also disturbed by the fact that her hands
and feet are often cold and sweaty.

These are all-too-familiar early symptoms of rheu-
matois arthritis. I have heard them told again and again,
and I know I can help.

But I worry when a new patient begs: "Say it isn't
so, tell me it is not rheumatoid arthritis!" In one way or
another—directly or only by suggestion—many patients
will ask for or even demand an opinion that I could not

34

possibly make until after I have done a general examination, seen the results of blood and other laboratory tests, and examined the X-rays of the affected joints. And even then, when all the first findings are at hand, I will still need to examine the patient repeatedly before I can be absolutely sure that this is, in fact, rheumatoid arthritis.

Nevertheless, many patients want some sort of instant verdict. When I am asked for this, I know I have a double duty to perform. Before I can help the patient fight her disease, I must first calm her fears and dread of rheumatoid arthritis; then, I can proceed to educate her.

I am always completely candid and truthful with my patients. There is an old Italian proverb that states, "He is not an honest man who has burned his tongue and does not tell the company that the soup is hot." So do not expect me to tell you that rheumatoid arthritis is a simple matter and that I have a secret method that will guarantee a cure. That would be deceitful and cruelly destructive. And, right from the start, I also feel obliged to educate the patient about my responsibility to her and her responsibility to me. We are in this together; it is an unsigned contract, a mutual commitment to do something positive about rheumatoid arthritis.

WHAT TO EXPECT FROM YOUR DOCTOR

The capable physician will approach rheumatoid arthritis as a long-term, chronic problem, not as an acute emergency. He will ease pain and discomfort, but he will promise no quick cure or complete control of symptoms. Instead, he will emphasize an extended program that consists of resting the joint or joints affected by rheumatoid arthritis, of the use of heat, and of specific exercises; he will prescribe a drug; if needed, he may suggest special counseling, be it psychological, rehabilitative, or vocational; also, some specific physical therapy, or even surgery.

If this seems undramatic, then let me point out that the past three decades have brought a number of major improvements in the care of rheumatoid arthritis patients. The most important, perhaps, has been the realization, based on scientific proof, that the conservative approach is enormously effective. We do not need new methods as much as we need to apply what we now know more widely and more effectively!

Conservative treatment comes first because it is the most helpful, and also the least hazardous, approach. It makes sense to try first what already has proved itself. Brand new or untried medications, especially, should be avoided. Too many of them share the curious history of cortisone, first used in 1949 and hailed as the "final" cure for arthritis. Soon enough cortisone proved too harmful to be used routinely; the risk posed by arthritis or any disease has to be great to justify any potentially hazardous treatment.

A doctor will do his best to control the symptoms. To suppress inflammation, he may take fluid from a severely swollen joint to ease the pressure (this is known as aspiration), or he may inject the joint with a drug to ease the pain. But that may be the extent of his emergency care. He will concentrate on a sound and safe basic program that he will re-evaluate at regular intervals. The doctor may want to see his patient weekly or every ten days at first, then every month or every three months; eventually, every six months may be enough.

Before a physician turns to more dramatic treatment, he wants to make sure that the basic approach has been understood and is being followed by his patient. Disability, even crippling, can result if his instructions are not followed faithfully. Perhaps the fact that conservative measures seem too simple is a major stumbling block. A patient's attitude is often the strongest deterrent to treatment. If he regards rest, exercise, and taking aspirin as tame compared to a fellow arthritic's use of a new "miracle" drug, then the conservative program will fail, and the patient will be in considerable difficulty.

The truth of this was demonstrated by Dr. Donald D. Weir of the University of North Carolina at the International Congress of Rheumatology, held in Prague in October 1969. He studied comparable English and American rheumatoid arthritis patients and how they were treated. The British physicians tended to utilize conservative therapy more frequently, and for longer periods of time; their patients were less inclined to seek quack magical cures and more readily accepted physical limitations. Furthermore, the English rheumatoid patients consulted specialists in physical medicine and rheumatology more often than their American counterparts to help with the details of specific remedial exercises, and to help plan long-range treatment.

By contrast, the American patients wanted a quick cure or at least substantial control of symptoms. Their general practitioners tended to approach rheumatoid arthritis as an acute disease and sought to provide prompt symptomatic relief. Dr. Weir points out that if complete relief is not rapidly forthcoming, another physician or a quack is commonly consulted. Steroids (that is, cortisone derivatives) are used often and early, and "too frequently the long-term results are disastrous." Details of Dr. Weir's fascinating study will be more fully discussed in Chapter IX. His work has again demonstrated what knowledgeable physicians now realize: There is no substitute for conservative, long-range planning in rheumatoid arthritis care.

In most cases, the doctor will start a rheumatoid arthritis patient on a basic, conservative program and then makes certain this program is being followed conscientiously. He may alter the program slightly by prescribing additional aspirin (or switching to another drug); he may suggest additional rest or different exercises. The physician will not consider a more toxic drug or surgery until, after several weeks of conservative treatment, he is convinced that his patient is not improving. Patients should not regard these first weeks as wasted time. For the advantage of first trying conservative treatment is that when it works, it works very well, and may be all the rheumatoid arthritis patient ever requires.

The specific treatment for each patient is based on what the physical examination, X-rays, and laboratory tests reveal. As his three major objectives of immediate treatment, the physician seeks to relieve pain, to prevent or reduce disability or deformity, and to arrest disease by suppressing the inflammation. To achieve these objectives, a doctor may decide to do one or more of the following:

He may hospitalize you early in the acute stage of rheumatoid arthritis or during a flare-up. Ordinarily such episodes last from two to four weeks, rarely longer. Hospitalization not only assures rest of inflamed joints, but also helps to orient the patient and her family to the needed long-term therapeutic approach.

He may treat you in the office by aspirating a joint to remove the excess fluid that is part of the inflammation, or he may inject a drug directly into the joint. These are, at best, temporary measures. But they may allow a patient to care for her family or go back to work. These injections should not be repeated more than three or four times a year. Given too often, they may injure the joint.

He may call in a specialist in rheumatic diseases, a rheumatologist, to advise on other drugs such as gold salts which require considerable expertise; he may obtain a surgical consultation to discuss the removal of the joint lining. Such surgery, called a synovectomy, will quickly improve joint function and has been especially successful for impaired hand and knee joints. Some patients have had separate synovectomies of many affected joints.

ARE THERE TESTS FOR RHEUMATOID ARTHRITIS?

There are a number. Doctors will order several blood tests that can help in making a diagnosis. There is no single test that is 100 percent accurate or that by itself can establish the diagnosis. Perhaps the most frequent tests are those done to detect the level of rheumatoid factor, an antibody that circulates in the blood of many people with rheumatoid arthritis. There are various tests for rheumatoid factor; the latex fixation test, the sheep cell agglutination test, and the Bentonite test are the ones most often done.

Another useful test is called the sedimentation rate; it measures the speed of settling of red blood cells to the bottom of a small test tube. When chronic inflammation exists, the cells settle more rapidly than is normal. Rheumatoid patients almost always have fast sedimentation rates.

Blood counts are done when the patient is first examined, also at frequent intervals to judge progress or to look for side effects from drugs. The same is true of urine tests. Sometimes a doctor may wish to make an analysis of joint fluid which can be removed quite easily and painlessly by tapping the joint with a needle. Also, when called for, a biopsy may be done; a surgeon may remove a small piece of tissue from the joint in order to examine it under a microscope.

WHAT ABOUT THE FUTURE?

At the beginning of rheumatoid arthritis, there is no way of telling whether the disease will be severe or mild, whether it will last or stop, whether it will spare the joints or end up wasting and destroying them.

I want my patient to know all there is to know about these possibilities. The truth frees them from the unknown, nameless dread; it is also an essential part of effective therapy. It provides "patient power"—the determination to do something positive and to fight with all available weapons. All of us know remarkable people who were told that they would be hopelessly crippled, unable to walk or work, who by dint of their own efforts have proved doctors wrong. Their motivation came from the anger of being told that they were hopeless. Unfortunately, this kind of angry effort is rare. Most often, patients just give up hope. I find that telling patients the truth about their disease and that they *can* help themselves is by far the best way of mobilizing for the battle ahead.

At the beginning of the chapter, I cited what Aristotle said about educated men being as much superior to uneducated men as the living are to the dead. I would like to amend this by adding that educated patients can lead full, rich lives, even despite the handicap of a serious, chronic disease.

The "say-it-isn't-so" patient with her built-in despair and ignorance can be educated, fortunately. But it is tragic when such education comes too late. This, in essence, was the misfortune of a sweet young woman, a former patient.

Marlene Smith was 27 years old when she experienced her first symptoms of severe rheumatoid arthritis. There was no way to predict that eight years later she would be hospitalized, too ill to keep house. But let her tell it to you in her own words:

> When the doctor told me I had arthritis, I cried. My sister had it after her third child was born, and though it cleared up after six months of gold injection treatment, she had terrible pain. I was afraid because gold did not work for me and cortisone only helped some.
>
> At that time nobody told me about exercises and splints or heat to keep my joints straight. Sometimes I thought my arthritis would just go away. I'd have as long as a week when I could walk across the room as though there was nothing wrong with me, then my hands and feet and knees would swell and hurt so that I couldn't get up to walk.
>
> I got pretty discouraged, so I went to this chiropractor who said he could get me well, but it would take a long time. He worked on my spine and he told me to cut down the cortisone. I did, but at the end of the year I was worse than ever. He said that was the fault of the cortisone.
>
> I was very depressed when I read an ad from a certain clinic which said they had helped thousands. I wrote and asked them for references and got the names of three people I could write to. The answers I got from these people said they had gotten good results, so my husband and I borrowed the money and I went out for a six-week period, which is what the clinic staff said I'd need. It turned out to cost twice as much as they said it would.

The first thing they did was to make me come off the cortisone altogether, then they gave me spinal manipulations, colonic irrigations, radio wave, ultrasound treatments, massages and baths and put me on a no-meat diet. I had managed to walk into the clinic but at the end of the six weeks I was so sick and in such pain I could not leave. They told me I must stay for two more weeks, but even then they had to carry me out on a stretcher. Those last two weeks cost $400. All together my stay cost almost $900. It took us a long time to pay back the money we had borrowed. Up to about three months ago, I still got letters from the same clinic urging me to go back; they also wrote that if I could get three other arthritics to go they would send me a check for $5, or they would give me a lower rate when I came back.

After this experience I thought I would never try anything again. I was afraid to go back to the doctor because he would ask me why I was off cortisone. For about a year I just stayed home and tried to take care of myself. For three months I just sat in a chair. Finally our home broke up and I could not take care of my three children. The organization that helped find a place for them put me in touch with the Arthritis Foundation and sent me to the arthritis clinic at Seton Hall College of Medicine in Jersey City. Right now I still can't walk, but I have had an operation on one hip and I only hope that everything will turn out all right. I would not want to tell anybody with arthritis what to do, but I feel if I had been able to find out what I now know early enough, I'd never have gotten so bad. To me the important thing is to keep fighting because every time you let it go for a while it gets ahead of you. You can't help yourself then and it just cripples you up. I was careless about keeping splints on my hands and they got worse right away.

Treatment is a steady and, I have to admit, a sometimes depressing struggle, but I wish I had back the years I spent trying other things or just giving up.

At the time this was written, already someone else was caring for her children. In 1963, when I saw her at the arthritics clinic in Jersey City, she was already helpless and confined to a wheelchair. Her hips were deformed and she was unable to straighten her knees. There was so little strength left in her crippled hands that she was barely able to feed herself or comb her hair. At this point, surgery was the only hope. We began with her hip deformities; and surgery helped somewhat. Sad to say, she still can't do too much for herself, and remains in a nursing home. Although her testimony helped put the disreputable quack clinic out of business, this is cold comfort to a strong and courageous woman who fights on despite the overwhelming odds.

For a small percentage of patients—probably less than five percent—it may be difficult to prevent the ravages of rheumatoid arthritis. It is conceivable that Marlene was one of them. Since she received only inadequate early care, we will never know. But, even if little or nothing could have been done to help her, at the very least we could have spared Marlene the agony of not knowing what was happening. If nothing else, this knowledge would have helped her through those bitter, hopeless years. I feel certain, too, we could have eased a great deal of her pain. If surgery had been performed sooner, she might have retained far more function of her hands, legs, and hips. But this is idle agonizing.

THE GOOD FORTUNE OF MAY BARTON

Let me tell you about a more typical rheumatoid arthritis patient, May Barton, who came to see me three months after she noticed some typical symptoms of rheumatoid arthritis. The first thing she mentioned to me was her lack of knowledge about arthritis, and that she did not trust what her friends and relatives had told her. She expected help from me, since she intended to go on living just as she had been.

In just a few minutes in the office, May Barton showed me her contempt for any disease that might interfere with a life she enjoyed. Just from that I knew that May Barton would do well, no matter how severe her disease might be. For she had courage, and courage is knowing when to ignore fear. Fear is a far greater enemy than any disease.

As it turned out, May's rheumatoid arthritis was starting very much the way Marlene Smith had told me her disease began.

May had nodules at the elbow and a high concentration of the blood protein called rheumatoid factor; both are known to be associated wtih a relatively severe form of rheumatoid arthritis. This is important, since early treatment is different for such patients. For instance, gold injections, along with aspirin, are given because there is some evidence that, in the more severe forms of rheumatoid arthritis, two antirheumatic medications, instead of one, may provide a better outcome. As it turned out, May Barton at first did well on only one drug.

At her first visit, I told May that next time we would have a "teaching" session, and that this would take three or four hours. I promised to explain all about the nature and treatment of her disease.

FIRST, THE DIAGNOSIS

When I next saw May, I began by reassuring her about her symptoms, such as the morning stiffness that had kept her inactive for two hours after getting up. I explained that the involvement of many joints, particularly of her hands and feet, as well as the fatigue and the loss of strength in her arms and legs, were all part of the disease. I told her the truth also about a possible poor outcome, or unfavorable prognosis, that might result because we had observed the presence of both nodules and a high level (titer) of rheumatoid factor. I explained why she needed several kinds of laboratory tests and how I would use the sedimentation rate of her red blood corpuscles (the erythrocytes) as a rough guide to the extent of the inflammation of her joints. When first performed, this blood test provides a baseline reading from which to judge future improvement. I remember being pleased that, while May did not fully understand.the details of the laboratory tests, she appreciated their importance and was delighted to know that there was some objective way of judging whether or not she was improving.

We then went on to discuss the results of the tests performed during her first visit. I pointed out that one of the blood tests had revealed that she was anemic, and that she was not to be concerned, since this often occurred in rheumatoid arthritis. The anemia accounted for some of her fatigue; both would gradually improve during treatment.

At the first visit, I had removed some joint fluid from May's swollen knee. It proved to be thin and opaque, rather than thick and clear as fluid from normal joints. We reviewed the X-rays together. They, too, provided an unwelcome, even surprising, finding. For although May had had symptoms for only three months, there were already small erosions noticeable in the small bones of her hands. Again, a bad sign.

Finally, I explained to May that one finding, the presence of so-called LE cells in a blood smear, might suggest that she had systemic lupus erythematosus, an even more serious disorder (see Chapter VII). But while rheumatoid arthritis and lupus may begin in a similar fashion, with joint pain and swelling, there are several ways to distinguish between the two conditions.

Patients with lupus may also have kidney problems, a characteristic "butterfly" rash over the bridge of the nose, a low white blood cell count, or even a breakdown (hemolysis) of red blood cells that causes profound anemia and purple blotches of the skin. May had none of these signs. Therefore, I could consider her diagnosis to be rheumatoid arthritis and begin to explain her treatment.

THEN BEFORE TREATMENT—THE
TEACHING SESSION

During the afternoon of our second meeting May Barton and I had the opportunity to become acquainted. Both of us asked innumerable questions. This teaching session is always my first chance to really get to know a patient with whom I will be working for months and years to come. I wanted to learn many things, including how May felt about herself, her husband, her two children, her home.

Does she worry about her teenager's draft status? Such a worry may have an influence on the course of the disease, and I try to prepare the patient for this cause and effect possibility. In any case, talking about whatever troubles her may very well help May to cope with her problems so that these problems do not affect her disease.

I like to find out what a patient enjoys in life, rather than just what is bothering her. I do this as much for the patient as for myself. I discuss what I enjoy, such as my love of gardening or food, since a mutual interest gives us an even better basis for understanding one another. If nothing else, I want every new patient to know that I am a human being concerned about the health and welfare of another human being.

Most rheumatoid arthritis patients have four "first" questions that they usually ask during this teaching session. They are: Why me—what did I do? What causes my disease? Exactly what is rheumatoid arthritis? And, if I move to Arizona, would the warm, dry climate improve my condition?

WHY ME—WHAT DID I DO?

It is surprising that so many patients really and truly believe that something they did wrong is responsible for their condition. Patiently and repeatedly, I try to tell each patient that nothing she did could influence the appearance of her rheumatoid arthritis. Such a patient wants the doctor to tell her that the disease is a punishment for some sort of misdeed. By being assured that this is just not so, a patient will begin to face the facts of her disease more realistically, and, leaving guilt and fear behind, begins to take proper care of herself.

WHAT CAUSES RHEUMATOID ARTHRITIS?

No one knows. The long history of rheumatoid arthritis is cluttered with once new but now discarded theories that explain the cause of this complex disease. Unfortunately the discredited theories just don't simply vanish, they live on, mostly by word of mouth. So there are a lot of people, doctors included, who still believe in the focal infection theory—the belief that a chronic infection in the body was somehow responsible for causing rheumatoid arthritis. Many teeth were pulled and many gall bladders were needlessly removed in the wake of this erroneous theory. Penicillin and the other antibiotics helped to make hash of the focal infections theory, since the use of these drugs sharply reduced chronic infections. However, rheumatoid arthritis continued as before.

Since the truth about the cause of rheumatoid arthritis is not known, half-truths flourish: a "bad" diet, for instance, is often blamed—usually too much wheat or meat, never both, I notice. But that is nonsense. One type of food cannot be responsible for so complicated a disease. Even being overweight is not in itself anything but a contributing factor to a patient's discomfort.

That congenital (inborn) transmission is a factor makes a good deal more sense. A fascinating, recently reported study by Dr. Stafford L. Warren of the University of California at Los Angeles has shown that in mice a disease resembling rheumatoid arthritis can be transmitted experimentally from parent to offspring "unto the fifth generation." But while this is enlightening scientific research, its significance for you and me has yet to be determined. Any application of this and other valuable research to the treatment of patients is many years away. It does not matter *after* you develop an illness whether heredity or predisposition is a cause. What does matter is that current research into the cause of rheumatoid arthritis must be supported. For it is the only way we will ever learn the true cause of rheumatoid arthritis. Once it is found, then treatment may be changed accordingly. And possibly we may also learn how to prevent the disease. Currently, some scientists believe that directly or indirectly viral or bacterial infections are involved.

Others are of the opinion that a form of rejection phenomenon occurs. There are those who believe a combination of these events is responsible.

The rejection phenomenon in an altered form may occur in rheumatoid arthritis. This phenomenon is now well known because this is what happens when the body refuses to accept a transplanted organ, such as the heart. Essentially, the body rejects any foreign substance and attempts to destroy the "intruder" if it fails to "recognize" the invader as part of itself. This can happen whether the foreign substance is large, like someone else's heart, or microscopic like invading bacteria or viruses. White blood cells (lymphocytes) produce antibodies in response to such invaders.

In rheumatoid arthritis, an indirect type of rejection appears to take place. But instead of the body attacking a foreign substance, it turns against itself. Theoretically this happens because, somehow, antibodies fail to "recognize" the body's own tissues and begin to destroy them as if they were foreign invaders. No one knows why this happens. But this strange aberration of the body's immunity system is implicated in a number of complex conditions known as autoimmune diseases.

Immunologists, scientists who study how the body protects itself against disease by means of its immunity system, have no final or conclusive evidence that rheumatoid arthritis is one of the autoimmune diseases. Research is still being done to find out why and how antibodies become *autoantibodies* so that, in effect, they are deceived and turn against the body that they are supposed to protect. A possible proof of this theory and one practical application of this research to rheumatoid arthritis patients is the current trial of the same immunosuppressive drugs that immunologists give transplant patients. These drugs are still experimental and, therefore, not generally available to rheumatoid patients. But one immunosuppressive drug, cyclophosphamide, used cautiously and given only to severely ill rheumatoid arthritis patients who failed to respond to other drugs, has achieved considerable success in a small number of patients; these drugs will be discussed in some detail later.

What causes the rejection phenomenon in rheumatoid arthritis? Some investigators believe that a bacteria or virus is the trigger that causes antibodies to become autoantibodies. Acting as if they were foreign substances or antigens, the autoantibodies then attack the tissue, muscle, or cartilage of a joint and in the process release powerful lysosomal enzymes from sacs along the lining of a joint. Once released from their so-called suicide sacs, the lysosomal enzymes destroy connective tissue, cartilage, and bone, causing widespread inflammation and damage characteristic of rheumatoid arthritis.

A self-perpetuating process then takes over. Autoantibodies originally were produced because of some sort of trigger; they in turn cause the release of lysosomes, which in turn not only cause destruction but also trigger the production of more autoantibodies. The original trigger, whatever it was, is no longer needed, since a self-perpetuating cycle is now set up. This theory of events might perhaps explain why rheumatoid arthritis persists throughout a patient's lifetime.

But remember, this is only a very simplified version of a complex hypothesis on which a number of brilliant researchers have been working for some years—and about which too little has as yet been finally established. Dr. Gerald Weissmann of New York University, the rheumatologist who first proposed the role of lysosomes in rheumatoid arthritis, has pointed out that lysosomal enzymes themselves can produce arthritis. Dr. Weissmann has demonstrated this in animals. Many drugs used in rheumatoid arthritis, he believes, stabilize or influence the activities of lysosomes; among these drugs are aspirin, gold salts, steroids, chloroquine, and perhaps also the prostaglandins, hormone-like substances that are beginning to be studied as possible arthritis drugs. This effect of various drugs on lysosomes may explain why they are effective in the treatment of rheumatoid arthritis, and may lead to the preparation of other drugs that are capable of influencing lysosomal function.

An enormous amount of research has been done on the action of these drugs; some of it is theory, much of it is continuing laboratory investigations. This work is part of a considerable and promising amount of basic research, which is vital to progress in understanding what occurs in rheumatoid arthritis, so that eventually new methods can be applied to the care of patients.

Emotions are also believed to cause rheumatoid arthritis. But this, too, has not been proven. Specialists in the field accept the active part played by anxiety, tension, or depression in aggravating existing disease in some patients. Many who are afflicted with rheumatoid arthritis have reported that the beginning of their symptoms either coincided or followed an emotional crisis or a distressing event, a death in the family, or some sort of separation, such as a divorce or a young son going into the army.

The reason I am so interested in the personal lives of my patients is that I have found that when emotional stress is relieved, or its influence on the disease understood, then improvement usually occurs. But I would not suggest a cause and effect relationship between rheumatoid arthritis and psychological problems.

WHAT IS RHEUMATOID ARTHRITIS?

When May Barton asked me this question, I answered, "I'm still learning. I hope I live long enough to really understand all about this long, complex, and difficult disease. But whether I ever do depends on others, on research investigators who are probing the mysteries of the cause of rheumatoid arthritis. My main concern is how my patients experience rheumatoid arthritis."

It is my aim, of course, to get my patients to experience their disease with a minimum of difficulties, pain, and discomfort. With their help and cooperation, this is possible for the overwhelming majority. Yet, patients are not alike. There is no standard form of rheumatoid arthritis. It may range from the hardly noticeable to the severely destructive. What I have learned from my patients is that in rheumatoid arthritis it matters less how severe your disease is than how the disease is handled. This is shown by Marlene Smith and May Barton who, it turned out, had very similar rheumatoid arthritis, but experienced their disease quite differently. Still, here are basic facts about rheumatoid arthritis that all patients need to know.

When it is severe, rheumatoid arthritis is the most painful and potentially the most crippling of all the major forms of arthritis. It is a chronic inflammatory disease, primarily of the joints—the knees, elbows, hips, hands and feet, or wherever two bones join to articulate. It also attacks the body's supporting structures, the connective tissue, such as the cartilage or the muscles that are found in all parts of the body. Consequently, rheumatoid arthritis can affect major organs in the body, for example, the heart, blood vessels, and lungs. In a recent report, Drs. David M. Roseman, Melville Magida, and Bernard Rogoff of New York's Hospital for Special Surgery reported several heart abnormalities that did not correspond to known disease among arthritis patients whom they examined at their clinic. They noted that 51 out of 104 older patients (between the ages of 40 and 70) had "cardiac abnormalities compatible with rheumatoid heart disease." This observation does not mean that if one has rheumatoid arthritis one will inevitably get heart disease. It does, however, illustrate the nature of the disease: It is a generalized disease of the body—it affects the entire human system. This affliction is not limited to the bones or muscles, it involves the whole body, although this may never become manifest. This is why rheumatoid arthritis is such a puzzling and capricious affliction.

The disease strikes at three times as many women as men, most often during the prime or most productive years of their lives, between 20 and 45. Older women, men of all ages, and even very young children are stricken. The most recent estimates suggest that rheumatoid arthritis affects about five million Americans.

Symptoms

The most usual symptoms of the disease are pain, soreness, swelling and redness of joints, with stiffness and accompanying loss of motion. The soreness and stiffness are at their worst in the morning when one gets up; the discomfort lessens progressively as one moves about for a while.

Consult a doctor promptly if you have the following symptoms:

• Persistent pain and stiffness after getting up in the morning
• Pain, tenderness, or swelling in one joint
• Recurrence of these symptoms, especially if the pain, tenderness, or swelling affects more than one joint and is

accompanied by fatigue or unexplained exhaustion, unexplained weight loss, or slight fever.

The recurrence of these symptoms signals a major warning: You need medical care now. It is the nature of the disease to alternate acute discomfort with symptomless periods. This naturally lulls patients into believing that there is really nothing wrong with them. But repeated attacks are injurious, and must be treated. Because of the "hit-and-run" aspect of rheumatoid arthritis, far too many patients delay seeking medical care until they sustain some irreversible damage to the movement or function of a joint.

An ominous sign of impending severe arthritis is the presence of small, hard nodules, or "lumps" beneath the skin, usually at the elbow, but also at the wrists, heels, or on the fingers. These are known as subcutaneous nodules. Unlike small loose bodies or "joint mice" that occasionally may be felt in the knee, they move and may disappear. These nodules are found in one out of five patients, and usually at the body's pressure points—a bed-ridden rheumatoid arthritis patient, for instance, may develop nodules on the back. The presence of one or more nodules should be reported to your doctor, especially when they occur in a spot of the body he may have failed to examine.

Involvement of Joints

Rheumatoid arthritis can involve or affect any joint of the body, but it most often strikes the small joints of the hands and feet. The synovial membrane, the lining of a joint, normally produces a lubricant, the synovial fluid, that "greases" the joint and allows smooth movement without the friction of one bone scraping against another.

In rheumatoid arthritis, when the synovial membrane is inflamed, it begins to produce abnormally large amounts of synovial fluid. Joint swelling results. As the inflammation continues, the ligaments, tendons, and other supporting structures of the joint become weakened. Then, as the disease progresses, the inflamed synovial membrane begins to grow over the smooth cartilage (the gristle or white elastic substance attached to the bone surfaces that allows bones to move or articulate smoothly). Eventually, the cartilage becomes eroded or eaten away, and fibrous scar tissue is left in its place. Joint action is attacked, because of the interference with articulation—the movement of one bone against another. This is the beginning of limited function.

If inflammation is severe enough, the space between the joints may become bridged by bands of fiber-like tissue. Eventually, these bands may be replaced by dense scar tissue that causes the joint to become fused (or ankylosed) so that it is fixed in position and cannot be moved at all. Ankylosis or joint fusion is usually due to fibrous scarring within a joint, rather than because two bones "grow together." Therefore, surgery can remove the fibrous tissues that prevent joint motion. But it is better to prevent fibrous scarring by proper care, the use of medicines, exercises, and physical therapy. This should be done in the early stages of the disease, while the joint is only inflamed. Then, only a minimum of permanent damage is likely to occur.

It is unusual for all the body's joints to be affected at the same time. Various joints will show different stages of the disease. May Barton, for instance, suffered from involvement of her hands, wrists, elbows, neck, knees, ankles, and feet. But her hips and shoulders were spared.

Rheumatoid arthritis continues with "ups and downs," with flare-ups and remissions. It is quite usual, even for the patient with severe rheumatoid disease, to have weeks, months, or even years during which pain and stiffness hardly ever occur or are totally absent. These periods of "easing off" are called remissions; they are just as sudden and unexpected as an attack or exacerbation of symptoms.

An important variant of rheumatoid arthritis is called psoriatic arthritis. It usually begins with a rash at the scalp line. The tricky thing about this condition is that the skin rash may precede the arthritis. You should be aware that this combination of arthritis and eczema tends to run in families. Tell your doctor if someone in the family has psoriatic arthritis or if you have a rash of the navel or on the elbow, or if you have scaling of the scalp. This is important, since the skin condition may have disappeared at the time you consult a doctor about your arthritis.

Whatever the skin eruption, and there are thirty or more forms, the arthritis is of several kinds. In "classical" psoriatic arthritis, patients will have the skin rash, pitted finger- and toenails, and inflamed arthritis involving only the end row of finger and toe joints. X-ray of the hands will show narrowing of finger bones where the arthritis occurs.

More common than classical psoriatic arthritis is the "rheumatoid-like" form with a generalized arthritis of major joints and involvement of organs of the body (as seen in typical rheumatoid arthritis). There are two major differences, however: subcutaneous nodules and rheumatoid factor are notably absent. The absence of rheumatoid factor is what may alert the doctor to this variant of rheumatoid arthritis.

Psoriatic arthritis can be devastating and mutilating, causing rapid destruction of the joints and even the surrounding bones. This is called "arthritis mutilans." Its management has to be vigorous, and must concentrate on the care of the rash. For reasons that are not clear, effective clearing of the psoriasis is often accompanied by lessening of the arthritis. A dermatologist, a physician specializing in skin conditions, should be consulted to make certain that the rash is treated promptly and properly.

Does Rheumatoid Arthritis Ever Just Go Away?

Yes. It has been known to stop at any point of the disease process. Sometimes rheumatoid disease will go away and never return. This is believed to happen in one out of every five patients; it is an unexplained phenomenon that has been observed in most long-term studies of adult patients with the disease. This may occur with or without treatment.

THE REMISSION PHENOMENON

Another mysterious and unexplained remission occurs when a woman with rheumatoid arthritis becomes pregnant; she may be freed from her pain and discomfort as early as the first months of pregnancy, and certainly during the last three months. She generally feels better, finds herself moving about more freely, is less tired, and has almost no difficulties with pain and morning stiffness, and there may be no swelling of her joints.

But then after the baby is born, the old symptoms return, usually within a month, sometimes within several months. The remission is over.

4

444

There is no logical explanation of this phenomenon, although female hormones are thought to be involved. Rheumatoid patients enjoy their surcease of symptoms, but it is unthinkable and impossible to use being pregnant as a form of treatment. This perhaps far-out concept did lead to a major discovery, for it prompted the late Dr. Philip S. Hench of the Mayo Clinic to use an artificial hormone, cortisone, for rheumatoid arthritis. His reward was a Nobel Prize, since he was the first to show that cortisone did indeed suppress rheumatoid inflammation. But unfortunately, the drug, its derivatives, and successors proved a mixed blessing, since large amounts could be taken safely only for short periods of time.

The remission phenomenon has led investigators to try other kinds of treatment, but none proved successful. They include the use of blood from the umbilical cords of newborn babies, and blood from pregnant women or pregnant mares. Such experiments have now been abandoned as offering no further promise.

Some relief from rheumatoid symptoms has been seen in both male and female patients during an attack of jaundice. In contrast to the rapid relapse after pregnancy, a remission due to jaundice may last for months or for perhaps two to three years. Again, and despite ingenious efforts to unlock the secret of this remission phenomenon, nothing satisfactory has been produced. Efforts to copy the jaundice remission have consisted of giving bile products or a drug that is mildly harmful to the liver. While worthy, these attempts have been disappointing; but they do suggest the importance of comprehensive care. For, despite all our hopes, there appears to be no "miracle" drug on the horizon that can do the job by itself, that is, produce a remission.

There are some physicians who actually discourage their rheumatoid patients from having children. They reason that patients have enough difficulties with their illness without the additional time and efforts that they will inevitably have to devote to a baby. I don't agree. This must be an individual decision, based on many things, particularly the attitudes of the patient and her husband. At least, this has been my experience.

Edna Axelrod married late because she had been a victim of rheumatoid arthritis for eight years. She was now 33, and two years after she married Paul, she and her husband came to me to seek advice on having a child. Paul explained that Edna's mother lived with them, and wanted to help with the care of a baby. Since they were anxious to have a child, and had already made arrangements for additional help with the child's care, I agreed—they should have a child.

Edna enjoyed six months of remission while carrying the baby. She had a slight flare-up a month after the baby was born. I increased the amount of aspirin Edna was taking. This and additional rest brought her rheumatoid arthritis under good control. The child is now five years old and much loved. The mother's disease is under beautiful control. For this family, having a child proved to be a wonderful experience. For some families, this may not be so. Therefore, I urge my patients to discuss both their disease and the circumstances of their lives with me when thinking about having children.

What About the Pill?

Sporadic reports that oral contraceptives may trigger or worsen a rheumatic condition has made me very suspicious of the pill.

One oral contraceptive has been associated with an unexpectedly high occurrence of rheumatoid factor. What that means remains to be determined. Doctors Donald R. Kay, Giles G. Bole, and William J. Ledger of the Univer-

sity of Michigan Medical Center Rackham Arthritis Research Unit reported the occasional presence of blood
abnormalities in a small number of women on the pill.
They found LE (lupus erythematosus) cells and antinuclear antibodies, the latter, one of the family of autoantibodies. These abnormalities usually disappeared when the
patients stopped taking the pill. Since autoantibodies are
suspected of being involved in the development of rheumatoid arthritis and since the pill seems to cause the
appearance of these blood factors, it may be wisest for
the patient with rheumatoid arthritis to avoid taking the
pill. Also, many rather serious questions are being raised
about the long-term effect of oral contraceptives (see Bar-
bara Seaman's book, *The Doctor's Case Against the Pill*
[New York: Peter Wyden, 1969]). Contraceptive methods,
if necessary, need to be discussed with your physician.

I should add a few words about what patients tell me
about their sex lives. For many, the need to continue their
usual sexual relationships with their husbands is great.
So, whenever possible, I try to raise the subject with the
husband to reassure him that rheumatoid arthritis is no
reason to stop loving his wife as he did before. Most of
the couples don't need this reassurance. More often, I
must convince the wife that her disease is not aggravated
by intercourse. If she refuses her husband, and blames
her disease, then she is expressing a pent-up anger against
her disease, while also trying to punish her husband. I try
to get a patient to talk about this and, if necessary, have
her talk to a marriage counselor, a psychiatrist, or a social
worker. It is important to a rheumatoid arthritis patient
to keep on living, and loving, as she would without her
disease. Using the disease as a weapon against her husband and the rest of the family would, inevitably, only
increase her problems. Worry and emotion only aggra-

vate the disease and may trigger recurrences, so it is vital to resolve all such conflicts, if at all possible.

WOULD IT HELP TO LIVE IN ARIZONA?

Dr. Joseph L. Hollander of the University of Pennsylvania found that sudden changes in weather, increased humidity, and decreased barometric pressure often increase the aches and pains of many arthritis patients. Similar symptoms may not be felt as sharply when there is little change in the weather. Therefore, like many healthy people, some arthritis patients find it more agreeable to live where there is an even, warm, dry climate. However, many factors besides the climate influence rheumatoid arthritis. The problems of physical or emotional strain, financial insecurity, or separation from family and friends may far outweigh the possible advantages of moving to a more stable climate. Ideal climate does not and cannot take the place of any part of treatment, and this, frankly, is what some patients may have in mind when they ask this question. So move to Arizona, California, or Florida if it is convenient, but rheumatologists will assure you that this move does not mean you are escaping from the disease.

IDEAL CARE FOR THE RHEUMATOID ARTHRITIS PATIENT

Having answered May Barton's first questions, I went on to tell her the plans I had for the treatment of her disease. What follows is essentially what we talked about that afternoon. Because so much was said, I gave Mrs. Barton some Arthritis Foundation literature to take home and read. This allowed her to have all the information

at her fingertips, as every arthritis patient should have.
These pamphlets are available locally.

How Treatment Begins: Rest, Heat, Exercise, Medicine

Before treatment, a patient needs only to remember
two things: If you consult a physician and his diagnosis is
rheumatoid arthritis and he does not start you on rest,
heat treatments, exercise, and medicine that are carefully
fitted to your specific problem and personality, then you
are not receiving proper care. Find yourself a doctor who
will start you off right, one who will deal with your specific problems with pain, limited ability to move, your
weight, your strength, your age, and endurance. I deplore
doctor-shopping, but I encourage seeking the help you
need.

Sufficient Rest

Rest is an all-important part of treatment. The amount
of rest a rheumatoid patient should get depends on the
degree and severity of joint involvement and also on the
presence of complications.

For May Barton I suggested a half-hour nap or rest
period every afternoon so that she would not get overtired in the late afternoon. I also urged her to get nine
hours of sleep every night.

Complete bed rest is needed only by the acutely ill
rheumatoid arthritis patients, those who suffer from
fever, fatigue, pleurisy, or heart trouble. A short stay in
the hospital is needed by other patients only if they can't
get physical and mental rest at home. There is much to be
said against complete bed rest: It is rarely needed and
may actually be harmful. So don't go to bed and stay
there just because you have rheumatoid arthritis. A
recent study revealed no advantage for complete bed rest

over unrestricted activity, that is, a balance between rest
and as much activity as a patient wanted.

Too much rest in bed may possibly lead to stiffened
and weak joints—just the opposite of what you and your
doctor want to achieve. And there are other complications of lengthy immobility—pressure ulcers (actually,
open wounds in the areas where you press against the
sheets), kidney stones, thinning of bones (osteoporosis),
loss of muscle mass and tone, and even the danger of
developing a blood clot in the legs.

When complete bed rest is needed, don't stay at home.
It is almost impossible to rest completely there. Go to a
hospital or sanitarium where there is someone to care for
you and to see that "bed-rest complications" are prevented. Joint and muscle movement will be maintained in
the hospital by massage and a certain amount of "passive"
exercise (when a therapist, nurse, or attendant moves
your legs and arms for you so that the joints are exer-
cised). I generally disapprove of passive exercises except
for an acutely ill patient.

At night in bed, try to lie as flat as possible; don't prop
your neck and knees with pillows. Don't use pillows
under the knees, for you will flex these joints and then
have difficulty straightening them out. A small pillow
may be used under the head, but don't overdo that either.

Strange as it may sound, sandbags and footboards have
been very useful for some patients. Let me explain why.
Your feet generally tend to turn out when you lie on your
back. This puts needless strain on knee joints which hurt
because of swelling and inflammation. To see that the
knee joints are properly rested, sandbags may be placed
along the outside of the feet; this keeps them from turning sideways and outward. Sometimes, the feet tend to
turn inward from the weight of bedcovers that may also

be too heavy for sensitive, swollen feet. The use of a foot-board or a simple frame from eight to twelve inches high will keep sheets and blankets sufficiently elevated.

Rest for the Joints—The Use of Splints

Fiberglass and other plastics have revolutionized splinting. Gone are those heavy, cumbersome plaster casts that patients used to dread putting on. Today, a patient wearing a lightweight splint can work around the house or continue working in an office. The other day I was in a stationery store where I was waited on by a saleslady who was wearing a splint to rest her right wrist. She was working, yet "resting" her wrist. That is the sensible way to use a splint.

The new materials used for splints are strong, light-weight, easy to fit accurately, and comfortable. Splints are used for both night and daytime "resting." Furthermore, a patient can put on and take off a splint by himself.

Splints are used when joints ache. Repeated splinting in a "functional" position—in which joints are straight, not bent—rests joints, preserves their function, and, most important, prevents possible deformity, since a painful hand, for instance, will be kept flexed to ease the pain. The result will be a flexion deformity, with the painful hand remaining frozen in the unnatural position assumed temporarily to ease pain. Splints are required when a joint is acutely inflamed, red, and painful, and continues to be that way despite several days of taking specific medicine to reduce the inflammation.

It is important to remember that an acute inflammation of a joint and with it the need for splinting occurs only once in a while and usually lasts from ten days to a maximum of four weeks, rarely for up to three months.

Resting an acutely involved joint by the use of splints is a necessary part of the total rest regimen required by many rheumatoid arthritis patients. Patients with a mild attack may need up to four hours of splinting during the day, in addition to a good night's sleep while wearing the splint. Ordinarily, patients do not wear more than two splints at a time, although sometimes one knee and two wrists might be splinted at the same time. I have found that patients quickly adjust to splints and regard them as only a minor inconvenience in view of their great advantage—for splints allow patients to keep active, moving, and even perhaps working.

The splinting "rest" program must continue even if painful joints at first continue to feel stiff after rest periods. Patients often mistake this as a sign that rest and splinting are not helping, and they will try to shorten or stop their prescribed rest time. But if they continue their program of balanced rest and exercise, they find that the stiffness and pain eventually diminish. The benefits of splints appear gradually.

Overture to Exercise: Heat to Tune Up the Joints

Hot or cold applications may provide some measure of temporary relief from joint aches and pains. They do not improve or change the basic arthritis. Try a cold compress or an ice bag (or ice cubes in a plastic bag wrapped in a towel) and notice its numbing effect where it is applied.

Heat treatment is far more popular, since it relaxes muscle spasm and limbers you up before you do your exercises. Everyone seems to have a favorite heat source, be it lamps, pads, compresses, tub or paraffin baths, or even diathermy, which a few doctors still use.

A warm tub bath is perhaps the simplest and most

effective way to apply heat to widely separated joints. But don't stay in water that is too hot for too long, since it may be exhausting. When you wish to heat only a small area of the body, soak a towel in hot water, then, after wringing it out, apply it to the painful joint. A sheet of plastic wrapped over the compresses will retain the heat longer.

I tend to feel that wet heat is a good deal more efficient than dry heat. Nevertheless, heating pads may be used, but only turned on low and for about 20 minutes. And nowadays heat pads for the hands, knees, elbows, and hard-to-reach places are available from "sleep shops" or specialty stores. You defeat the purposes of heat treatment if it is too long; more rather than less muscle pain and spasm will result.

For the small joints of the hands and feet, paraffin baths are a particular favorite of some of my patients. They put four pounds of paraffin wax and two ounces of mineral oil into the upper part of a three-quart double boiler, with plenty of water in the bottom section. They heat the wax until it melts, remove it from the heat, and allow it to cool. The wax is ready for use as soon as a thin white coating appears on top. Then, with fingers slightly separated, a patient dips one hand at a time in and out of the paraffin. This is repeated seven or eight times; each layer of wax is allowed to cool. The heat will be retained longer if someone helps you and wraps your hands in a towel or cloth. Or you can do this by yourself one hand at a time. Eventually the wax cools, cracks, and peels off cleanly, so it can be reused. Some of my patients do this daily and, once they get started, have found it a simple, inexpensive, and efficient physical measure.

But remember, whatever the source of heat you use, don't overdo it, and don't sustain burns. No heat treatment should last longer than the absolute maximum of 30 minutes.

Exercise as Treatment

Therapeutic exercises must be suited to the individual. This comes as a surprise to many of my patients, but they should know better. All athletes appreciate the fact that exercise is a science keyed to the job intended. For athletes, this most often means strengthening and building up a specific set of muscles. They turn to physical-fitness experts for help. The arthritis patient has a broader goal beyond strengthening muscles, and that is to maintain a normal range of motion and to prevent deformity. For this you need a physician to design a tailor-made set of exercises. In a hospital or medical center, this is done by the doctor who specializes in physical medicine, the physiatrist, or by his assistant, a physical therapist.

Therapeutic exercise is the least appreciated, yet perhaps the most important part of treatment of rheumatoid arthritis. Unfortunately, patients must be their own training coaches. While they have active disease, they must faithfully do prescribed exercises. Most people hate to exercise, and this is why its benefits are so little valued. But exercise may often make the difference between leading an active life and being crippled. Patients who overcome their natural reluctance to exercise soon become devoted converts.

My favorite example is Beatrice de Monteleone. Almost fifty years ago, the Countess Monteleone was told in Italy that she would become hopelessly crippled and spend the rest of her life in bed, because the joints of her hips and knees were rapidly beginning to lose their full function. But she was determined to keep limber and began exercising, to stretch and extend, to keep mobile. Now at 83, she still exercises, is still on the move, and seems to have outlived both her original doctors and any possible ill effects of rheumatoid arthritis. She exercises the way other people brush their teeth—it is part of her life. "It keeps me going," she confesses with a blithe smile.

Patients are often mistaken when they think they are exercising while working. Cleaning the house or other work activities may prove to be too strenuous. This may promote discomfort and even accelerate deformities.

For the severely ill patient with very active and hot arthritis of many joints, the early period of exercise may be limited to assisted exercises to provide the maximum range of motion to all major joints. Assisted exercises are done for the patient by a therapist or family member. However, most patients can and should do their own exercising.

Most are performed lying on the back, and all major joints are taken through their normal range of motion. At first, two or three repetitions of each exercise are to be done at least three times daily, in the morning, afternoon, and evening. Later, this has to be increased to ten or twenty repetitions of each exercise, three times daily. Each motion should be done slowly and deliberately in order to achieve the maximum range of motion wherever possible.

Special attention should be given to the big thigh and buttock muscles, because they tend to weaken rapidly, especially when a patient is inactive or in bed. Simple "setting exercises" should be done by contracting and then holding muscles tight for a few seconds; such isometric exercises are easy to do frequently during the day to maintain strength in important muscles.

When active or acute disease has diminished, a more vigorous exercise program should be begun. Expect some joint discomfort, especially after the more difficult exercises.

How much exercise can a patient do? There should be no greater pain an hour after the exercise is done. If exercises are followed within 24 hours by an increase of pain, swelling, or stiffness, this should be taken as a signal to cut down the physical activity. Too much exercising may cause a flare-up of a smoldering arthritis. Therefore, reduce or modify the amount, but do not stop. Remember, as improvement occurs, the amount and type of exercise will be changed.

Diet and Dieting

"Should I be eating something else than I am?" May Barton asked me. Somehow this question always arises during the lengthy teaching session, even though I already pointed out that diet does not influence the appearance or course of rheumatoid arthritis. Before I can sensibly answer the question, I need to know what a patient eats.

But even without this knowledge I can outline a few basic rules. The healthiest people are those who pay attention to themselves, what they do, and what they eat. I tend to think that the French proverb, "Death enters by the mouth," is picturesque but a little exaggerated; we do not really dig our graves with our teeth. Still, we all should eat a properly balanced diet, one adequate in calories, with a maximum of protein, enough vitamins and minerals, and a minimum of fat and starches. Everyone should also be aware that as they grow older they should reduce rather than increase the total amount they eat. This is repeatedly suggested by some leading nutritionists. Every ten years, eat ten percent less, they advise. This is easy to urge, and hard to do; but for the overweight rheumatoid patient, there is no alternative except to lose weight at once.

In my experience, however, most rheumatoid patients are underfed or poorly nourished because of their lack of appetite. So frequently early treatment includes a nutritional build-up.

Let me again stress that there is no diet that will either help or prevent the disease, any future attacks, or influence the outcome of the disease. And believe me, I have investigated this question to the best of my ability during the years I have been a rheumatologist. Many, far too many, of my patients are attracted to fad diets. Fortunately, they rarely stay on them long enough to do themselves any harm. But it does worry me when an otherwise intelligent person is even momentarily taken in by the nonsense that honey and vinegar will be of great benefit or perhaps even "cure" the disease. That is the type of error that Marlene Smith made. By itself, it may do little harm, but to substitute honey and vinegar for a sensible diet, and perhaps even for treatment, is very dangerous.

It is bitter to find out that a patient of mine would trust such folly. To me it means someone is giving up hope in herself and no longer trusts me. Then, I know, I must start all over to convince and educate.

Losing weight, too, may be a task in persuasion. And I try hardest with the occasional rheumatoid patient who has arthritis of the hip, knee, or any other weight-bearing joint. Actually once such a patient has lost weight, she needs no convincing. Mrs. Enid Roff is an example. I had much difficulty trying to get her to take off 25 to 50 pounds. She was unwilling to lose weight, since she doubted that this would really influence the progress of the disease. She had rather extensive hip involvement and, despite the fact that she was then over 70, we had discussed the possibility of hip surgery.

Some time passed during which I had not seen Mrs. Roff regularly. Then one day, I discovered her sitting outside my office. I asked her to follow me in. Although she was using a cane, I was amazed to see how fast she moved.

"You must be feeling a lot better," I said. "I'm really not sure," she answered. "The big difference has been the weight I've lost. Everyone has noticed how much quicker I am on my feet, and I realize I am moving faster. It has done wonders in making me feel comfortable, and I would like to lose more." And then, as she took off her coat, I realized that she had indeed taken off twenty-five pounds, and not only was it becoming, making her look younger, but it ultimately proved to be a sensible alternative to the surgery that had been suggested, but that she dreaded and refused to undergo.

The weight loss removed the pressure of excessive weight from a hip sufficiently troubled by pain and inflammation, and it will do the same for a knee, ankle, or any of the weight-bearing joints afflicted with arthritis. Gaynor Maddox, who wrote a diet handbook for patients with arthritis (available from the Arthritis Foundation), also has a book out on the subject that I recommend (*Food and Arthritis* [New York: Taplinger Publishing Co., 1969]). It contains over 150 menus and 125 recipes selected and tested by panels of arthritic homemakers. In words and pictures it also offers good advice on how to plan or remodel a kitchen so that the housewife with arthritis will reduce to a minimum the muscular strain and fatigue of meal preparation. Particularly helpful are the photos showing how a patient with limited use of her hands can open a can, slice a potato, grate a carrot, or reach for a container on a high shelf. A pamphlet called "Home Care in Arthritis," available from the Arthritis Foundation, contains a section on self-help devices, and lists helpful books and information sources.

MARVELS BUT NOT MAGIC: MEDICATIONS

I am often disturbed to find that even my most intelligent, cooperative, and well-motivated patients are completely confused about the limited usefulness of drugs in rheumatoid arthritis.

All patients pin disproportionately high hopes on the use of one or another of the antirheumatic drugs. But there are no drugs to cure the disease, only a number that will suppress joint inflammation, and only partially at that. Drugs—whether aspirin, gold salts, cortisone and its derivatives, or any of the newer agents—are only a small part of complete care. Drugs cannot take the place of the other necessary forms of treatment—rest, heat treatment, exercise, or other physical measures. When they do, patients are in trouble. Drugs can be marvelous, but they offer no magical solution. They serve primarily to ease the pain so that the patient can comfortably begin a program of exercise.

And let me advise all rheumatoid arthritis patients that if they now have a doctor who prescribes a drug and does nothing else for them, they are not in good hands. I would like them to find a physician who sees the usefulness of drugs in proper perspective as only a part—although a vital one—of total care.

When it comes to explaining about drugs, I find that I spend a disproportionate amount of time defending the use of aspirin. Despite doubts by patients, this is the first and logical choice for treatment. It is the least harmful and most effective drug available for rheumatoid arthritis. Only if it proves ineffective should another drug be considered. This is sound, conservative therapy. Patients may feel "cheated" to be told that they have a serious disease and then are given a prescription for aspirin. May Barton expressed some reluctance about taking aspirin until she learned more about this unique and versatile 71-year-old "miracle drug." Today aspirin is used in more than a thousand products and consumed in staggering quantities—an estimated 35 million pounds in the United States alone.

In an informative article in *The New York Times Magazine*, George A. W. Boehm pointed out that while "generations of patients dosed with antibiotics, hormones, mood regulators and other fearfully potent medications may regard aspirin with some contempt, medical scientists respect it highly. It is, to be sure, cheap, easy to get—and disarmingly safe . . . Indeed were it invented today, aspirin would be hailed as a wonder drug because of its versatility."

Why Aspirin?

Because it is the "first line of defense" in treating rheumatoid arthritis, according to Dr. Charley J. Smyth, head of the Rheumatic Disease Division of the University of Colorado School of Medicine, one of the leading experts on drugs used in arthritis.

As recently as 1958, Dr. Russell L. Cecil, one of the most distinguished arthritis specialists of his day, wrote that aspirin has "little more than an analgesic effect on the rheumatoid patient." Scientists have discovered much about aspirin since 1958. Analgesia or the alleviation of pain is only one of the three basic actions of the drug. Aspirin also reduces fever and, most important for the rheumatoid arthritis patient, it suppresses joint inflammation.

In recent years this property of aspirin has been repeatedly confirmed in large-scale trials by the American Rheumatism Association in the United States and in England by the Medical Research Council. So don't downgrade aspirin; it is and remains the most valuable of antirheumatic drugs, the most frequently used medication in rheumatoid arthritis. In 1966, the *Newsletter* of the Northern California Chapter of the Arthritis Foundation figured out how many aspirin tablets are being taken in this country every day. Their estimate is 1,184,000,000! Over a billion a day! I suspect that the number is even larger. "If you are taking aspirin for your aches and pains you have a lot of company," the *Newsletter* concludes.

However, to be effective in suppressing inflammation, aspirin *must* be taken in sufficiently large doses. The daily dosage will range from 12 to 24 five-grain tablets.

You, together with your doctor, will determine what amount of aspirin you should take. The largest tolerated amount is what should be taken in rheumatoid arthritis to the point where your ears begin to ring, a condition known as tinnitus. Then you will also be able to tell whether the aspirin is helping you. Your doctor can use objective measurement of the size of a swollen finger; but so can you. If the wedding ring you have had difficulty slipping off your finger goes on and off smoothly, then the drug is working to reduce inflammation and swelling.

When a patient tells me that aspirin has not helped, then I try to discover whether she has actually taken the amount I suggested.

Often I am able to solve the problem by a little detective work. Too frequently, a patient will simply not take enough aspirin. I customarily start prescribing three five-grain tablets every four hours at least five times a day. Some patients must set the alarm in order to take a sixth or night-time dose. Then we start adjusting the dosage— often settling for 15 five-grain tablets daily. It usually does not take too much sleuthing to find out if all the tablets have really been taken, or if a dose has been over-looked. If this has happened, then I explain the vital importance of all those tablets. First of all, the rheumatoid patient must achieve *high* levels of aspirin in her blood. For aspirin to be effective, it must constitute from 150 to 250 milligrams (mg.) of every liter (roughly a quart) of blood. Such saturation will ease the pain and reduce the rheumatoid inflammation.

Another reason that so many tablets are needed to help the patient with rheumatoid disease was found by Drs. Theodore B. Bayles and Kenneth Fremont-Smith of Harvard Medical School. They have shown that the rheumatoid patient with active disease needs almost double the amount of the drug to achieve high aspirin blood levels than does a patient with inactive rheumatoid disease, an osteoarthritis patient, or a person without arthritis. Perhaps when this finding is better understood, specialists will know more about the nature of the disease. At this time, all I can do is to urge my patients to take the full amount—and do not think that fewer aspirins won't make any difference. They do. The chief reason that aspirin is too quickly abandoned or found valueless is that insufficient amounts are being taken.

Brand preferences may cause even more tricky problems. To resolve this dilemma, I advise patients to take the type of aspirin that they tolerate the best. I favor a buffered product. Let me explain why.

The original of what we now know as aspirin is salicylic acid. It is a substance abundantly found in nature, for instance in the bark of the willow tree or in a genus of shrubs, the spiraea. What we take in tablet form is a chemically produced substance, a synthetic product. Unfortunately, pure synthetic salicylic acid is irritating to the stomach, while a chemical modification, sodium salicylate, has a taste so sweet as to make one nauseous.

The form of salycilate used in all aspirin preparations is acetylsalicylic acid. This is exactly what Friedrich Bayer & Co., the German chemical company, introduced in 1899. Later they produced a tablet consisting of acetylsalicylic acid compressed with a little starch. It was Bayer who dubbed their product aspirin, a combination of the words "acetyl" and "spiraea," the salicylate-rich type of bush. The name aspirin was the exclusive trademark of Bayer until just after World War I, when a U.S. court denied the company's rights to the name; it was then that the trademarked "Aspirin" became generic "aspirin," and the name is now universally used for any and all forms of acetylsalicylic acid.

The problem with aspirin is that it is slow to dissolve, and as it does, it may irritate the lining of the stomach. As noted before, aspirin must be absorbed by the blood from the stomach in order to exert its benefits. Work continues on less irritating and more quick-acting aspirin. But, so far, none has been produced. What are the alternatives? There are several, fortunately.

I recommend Bufferin, a product of Bristol-Myers. Aluminum salts are included in this aspirin product, and as some research of mine has demonstrated, these salts do reduce irritation and help speed absorption of the aspirin into the bloodstream. Another plus of this product is that it contains the full five grains of aspirin that are the basis of all my prescriptions.

Many other aspirins currently on the market are combinations of aspirin and other standard pain-killing products. Most often they consist of six parts aspirin, three parts phenacetin, and two parts caffeine. Because phenacetin was found to be harmful to the liver when taken for long periods of time, some of these products now no longer contain it in their formula and substitute other ingredients (salicylamide or ammophenol). Products still including phenacetin post a warning on each bottle. Such combination products may confuse the consumer. Also, not all these products contain the full five grains of aspirin; some have only three grains. Therefore I advise use of the buffered aspirin. There is no real scientific support of the claims that combination products are any better than aspirin alone. Eventually, no doubt, an effective, speedy, and long-acting product that releases aspirin gradually over a full eight-hour period will be produced. One such medication was withdrawn from the market some years ago because the Government felt excessive claims had been made for it.

Aspirin is generally harmless, despite its tendency to cause stomach discomfort. There is an occasional patient who is unable to take even the buffered product. These people are so sensitive to aspirin that a single tablet may cause a severe, perhaps even fatal, asthma attack. I do not prescribe aspirin for patients with peptic ulcers, or those who are taking a medication that thins the blood (anticoagulants).

Tell your doctor if you have ever experienced any trouble with aspirin. Together, you can decide if these are minor difficulties that may be overcome, or sufficiently severe to prevent your taking the drug.

To minimize the stomach-upsetting capacity of aspirin,

I suggest taking the tablets with milk or just after meals. Do not take aspirin on an empty stomach, and never without water or some other liquid.

Only if aspirin really proves ineffective will I consider another drug in addition to it or in its place. Unfortunately, there is no way to tell which patient will best respond to or benefit from what drug. Therefore, several drugs may have to be tried, either singly or together. These added or alternative medications include indomethacin (Indocin), phenylbutazone (Butazolidin), antimalarials, gold salts, and the cortisone derivatives, the adrenocorticosteroids. Here, briefly, is what you should know about each of them.

Indocin

If aspirin does not work, Indocin may be considered next, even though its value in rheumatoid arthritis remains a matter of debate. This relatively new drug has been given together with aspirin, but recent investigation suggests that when these two drugs are taken together they may compete with another. But whether they cancel out each other's effectiveness remains to be demonstrated.

The initial dosage of Indocin is usually one capsule (25 mg.) given two or three times a day, preferably right after meals and with a bedtime snack to lessen gastrointestinal upset. The dosage can be increased during a two-week period until six or even eight capsules are taken. But this amount may be risky, since side effects of the drug tend to be more extensive at higher dosages, and include nausea, vomiting, diarrhea, dizziness, and morning headache. The headaches often disappear while the drug continues to be taken.

Indocin should not be given to children, pregnant women, or easily excitable "over-reactors." The psychologic after-effects of Indocin may appear gradually—the housewife is more than usually depressed and unhappy, while a male patient may complain that he is not as alert at work as he formerly was.

If after two weeks, Indocin has not made an appreciable difference in symptoms, then another drug should be tried.

Butazolidin

Because of its possibly toxic effects on bone marrow and kidneys, this drug should only be taken for short periods of time. Bimonthly blood counts must be done, and also tests of the urine, to make sure no changes are taking place that may be harmful. The most efficient use of Butazolidin is during a flare-up of rheumatoid arthritis, when it is used for less than four weeks. It may be given in addition to aspirin.

The daily maintenance dosage of Butazolidin is three or four tablets (300 to 400 mg.). Like Indocin, Butazolidin should be discontinued if within two weeks no improvement occurs. There is virtually no difference between Butazolidin, Butazolidin-alka, which contains antacids to reduce stomach irritation, and Tandearil, a newer form of this drug.

The Antimalarials

Occasionally, these drugs may prove to be effective in patients who do not respond to any other medication. But they have two major drawbacks—a delayed action and some serious side effects. It takes from two to eight weeks before these drugs begin to work. Antimalarials are used cautiously by physicians, who urge their patients to be on the alert for symptoms of eye changes—fuzzy vision or halos around lights—that precede serious difficulties. If an antimalarial drug is chosen by your doctor, he should also insist that you see an ophthalmologist every six months just to make sure that no symptomless eye problem is developing. These drugs do not affect just the pigmentation of the eyes; they are also likely to cause skin or hair color to change or lighten when the patient is exposed to the sun.

Despite these potential dangers, there are some doctors who are extremely skillful in the use of these drugs, and their patients appear to do very well.

The Gold Salts

Gold salts are thought to be especially helpful during the early phases or first year of rheumatoid disease. These injections are regarded by many physicians as a measure of last resort to be given only by arthritis specialists. But even the rheumatologists are not in full agreement about the usefulness of gold therapy. One of the major stumbling blocks is that one cannot predict which patients will respond to gold. Also, like the antimalarial drugs, gold takes a long time before exerting any beneficial effects.

Generally, a positive response takes from three to six months of weekly injections. The weekly dose is about 50 mg. until approximately 800 to 1,000 mg. have been injected. Then the interval between injections becomes longer until only monthly injections are necessary. These are continued as long as they are of benefit and no side effects are encountered. But there may be both major and minor complications attributable to the gold salts—skin rash, a metallic taste that precedes ulcerations (or sores) of the mouth, kidney problems, or blood disease. Since some of these complications of treatment are serious—and in the case of blood disease, potentially fatal—it is vital that blood and urine tests monitor a patient's progress. Despite all these reservations, or perhaps because I am so aware of them, I have managed to treat hundreds of patients successfully with gold salts.

Cortisone—First the Dazzle, Then the Disappointment

"Probably no disease has been subject to so many 'breakthroughs' and so many promises of 'cures' in the public press than has rheumatoid arthritis," *The Medical Post*, a Canadian publication for physicians, recently pointed out. The newspaper was citing the optimism expressed by two distinguished rheumatologists, Dr. Donald F. Hill of Tucson and Dr. Ephraim P. Engleman of San Francisco, about treating rheumatoid patients even though they stressed that in treating this disease "one cannot think of short-term goals. In spite of the importunities of the patients, goals which give early, short-term relief (such as those obtained by the steroids) are not in the best interest of the patient. Results are to be considered in terms of five, ten, or 20 years."

Those wise words come just two decades after a thrilling future was forecast for cortisone, the mother drug of all the steroids. Cortisone, it was claimed, was the answer —the seeming solution to the problem of rheumatoid arthritis. Though the cause of the disease was unknown, the "cure" was at hand! Sadly, it was a matter of claiming in haste, and withdrawing the boasts at a snail's pace. For many patients it was a matter of going from apparent medical "breakthrough" to personal heartbreak. But then, the more fervent the hope, the slower its death. Nonetheless, this is only part of the story. There is also much good to be said for the steroids.

"Few clinical discoveries in the history of medicine have had such a profound influence on medical research . . . as has the observation that cortisone can reverse the inflammatory changes of rheumatoid arthritis," Dr. Roger L. Black of the National Institutes of Health has observed. And actually, this is mild praise for a drug whose derivatives and successors have, within a relatively short period of time, found their place in more than fifty ailments of man. Called variously adrenocorticosteroids, glucocorticosteroids, corticoids, steroids, or by their generic names—cortisone, hydrocortisone, prednisone, dexamethasone, etc.—these are all variations of a group of hormones essential to life.

The word steroid derives from the Greek *stereos,* solid, and the Latin for oil, *oleum.* Everyone is acquainted with the most familiar "solid oil," cholesterol, a sterol, to which the steroids (substances resembling sterols) are closely related. Both are built on a common chemical framework, the steroid nucleus. Among the important steroids are male and female sex hormones and hormones of the bark or cortex of the adrenal glands (which perch directly on top of the kidneys).

Cortisone was the first adrenal steroid to be used medically, after its powerful anti-inflammatory activity was first demonstrated by Dr. Philip Hench and his associates at the Mayo Clinic. Synthesized or man-made cortisone-like compounds are generally called corticoids; they were produced by various drug companies to be more specific, effective, and less injurious. It is curious that these drugs continue to be among the most widely used in the world, even though their use in rheumatoid arthritis, as well as in other rheumatic diseases, has been increasingly criticized. In 1969, the prestigious National Academy of Sciences–National Research Council warned that the risk of steroids in rheumatic disease often outweighs the advantages of disease suppression. The 30-man panel had made a thorough investigation of some 4,000 preparations and investigated 10,000 therapeutic claims made for these drugs. In their report to the Food and Drug Administration, they noted that "a considerable number" of the drugs examined were effective for all claims made for their use. But almost ten percent did not live up to all claims made, and a great many of the drugs were found useful in the treatment of some but not necessarily all the conditions they claimed to help.

This report is merely part of the sobering reappraisal being made of many old and new drugs about which we seem to know too little.

For the steroids, the consensus of opinion among qualified workers appears to be that they should rarely be the first drug in the treatment of a patient with rheumatoid arthritis.

Steroids should only be given after a thorough and unhurried trial of conservative measures, including the least harmful drugs. Only if these fail should steroids be considered. And then, before starting a patient on steroids, a careful search must be made for any possible infection or other factors about the patient or the disease that might oppose or contraindicate the use of such potent agents.

In any case, steroids are not to be used alone. Like any other drug, they cannot constitute the only form of treatment for rheumatoid arthritis. They must be part of a comprehensive and individualized treatment program.

May Barton had, of course, heard about steroids. But like many patients she knew only of their remarkable advantages. She had never heard of the side effects—such as peptic ulcers, Cushing's syndrome with the moon face and growth of beard on women, thinning of the bones known as osteoporosis and spontaneous fractures that result, or psychosis, diabetes, obesity, lowered resistance to infection—the list is long and frightening—that make these drugs so dangerous.

Steroids should be used only if nothing else works. A patient must be informed of the risks involved—principally that after taking these drugs for more than six months, it may be difficult or even impossible to stop taking them. The longer someone takes a steroid and the larger the dosage, the more difficult is the eventually necessary "weaning" process. "Withdrawal" is easier if a patient takes only small doses for less than six months. But even if small doses are taken, the normal adrenal function may be altered. For up to two years after steroid therapy has been discontinued, even patients who have been taking small doses for less than six months must carry a card stating that in case of accident or infection, they will require steroids for a few days to enable them to sustain or even survive the physical stress of illness or injury.

Despite all these dangers, and despite the many frequent warnings about the hazards of these drugs, far too many doctors are still using steroids far too freely. They, too, need education. This was shown in the 1966 poll on medical practice, conducted by a famous professional publication, *Modern Medicine*. The magazine wrote 11,603 doctors, of whom 5,694 answered. Half were general practitioners, more than a quarter internists, and the rest specialists, such as surgeons, pediatricians, physiatrists. They were treating 104,010 patients. What emerged from the poll was that the general practitioner, the internist, and the surgeon were giving steroids to about half of their patients. My educated guess is that steroids should not be used in fifty percent of patients, but perhaps in less than twenty percent.

Steroid Injections

So far, my discussion of steroids has centered about drugs taken internally for their systemic effect. The warnings and precautions about the steroid medications you take by mouth do not hold true for those a doctor injects into a joint.

The removal of fluid from a joint (joint aspiration) and the intra-articular injection of steroids have a definite role in the treatment of rheumatoid arthritis. If large amounts of synovial fluid are causing joint pain, aspiration alone may bring relief. When a patient has one or two joints that are much more severely affected than some others, I frequently try aspiration and then give a steroid injection. The effect achieved is often remarkable. Within a few days, the pain and discomfort are gone and this relief may last for months or more, depending on the drug and the dosage. However, a "post-injection flare-up" may occur within 24 hours, so that the injected joint becomes more painful until the flare-up subsides, within a day or two.

There is a little risk involved in giving these injections; very rarely a hemorrhage might develop or the injection might be the cause of an infection. Weekly or monthly injections cannot be given because this would threaten the bone. Therefore, steroids should not be injected more than two or three times a year.

Immunosuppressive Drugs

At the end of the line of useful drugs are several anti-cancer agents. They are used only in a small portion of brave human "guinea pigs" who, unfortunately, have no other choice but to take the considerable risks involved. But, then, they are the most tragic of the rheumatoid arthritis patients, those with severe and unrelenting disease.

Dr. William M. Fosdick of Tucson told the December 1969 meeting of the American Rheumatism Association (ARA) about one of these drugs. "The known risks and possible as yet unknown side effects of long-term therapy with [the drug)] require that it still be reserved for patients suffering from severe, active disease which is resistant to all conventional therapy."

Dr. Fosdick was talking about cyclophosphamide (Cytoxan), but what he said holds true for the other immunosuppressive drugs. He reported encouraging results—95 of his 108 rheumatoid patients were benefited, 29 were in complete remission, having no disease, the rest were improved, with 45 in partial remission confirmed by laboratory tests, while 21 showed evidence of remission that could not be confirmed by laboratory tests. Thirteen patient failed to respond.

Dr. Donald Mainland of New York University Medical Center reported to the ARA meeting on the results of a cooperative study of this drug, sponsored by the association and now in process at a number of clinics. He stressed the importance of "very frequent and systematic observations of patients on Cytoxan." The study, he felt, did not reveal all the potential dangers of this drug. "The work of others has shown that administration of the drug, especially when prolonged, has been associated with death from various causes, namely hemorrhagic cystitis, the unloosing of infections, such as mycoses [fungus infections] and disseminated acute infections, both viral and bacterial." Ovarian suppression and teratogenesis (the production of a malformed child) are also potential hazards. This, again, applies to the rest of the group of these drugs.

The first immunosuppressive drug used experimentally to treat rheumatoid arthritis was mechlorethamine (Mustargen), also known as nitrogen mustard. Introduced commercially by Merck in 1950, the drug is currently used to treat leukemia, lymphosarcoma, Hodgkin's disease, and other forms of cancer. After repeated clinical tests in patients with rheumatoid arthritis, beginning in the early 1950s, the drug was finally rejected for treating this disease because of its many adverse side effects.

In recent years, other immunosuppressive agents have been tested in arthritis patients. Among these are 6-mercaptopurine (Purinethol), chlorambucil (Leukeran), azathioprine (Imuran), cyclophosphamide (Cytoxan), cytosine arabinoside (Cytarabine), and methotrexate (Methotrexate, formerly known as A-methopterin).

The overriding problem with all these drugs is that they can block a large part of the body's immune response, knocking out the body's defenses against infection. Thus, a patient taking such a drug may become readily susceptible to pneumonia, tuberculosis, or to other infectious diseases.

These drugs can damage or destroy bone marrow, and affect the formation of almost all types of white and red blood cells, as well as blood platelets. White cells are among the body's principal means of combating infection, while blood platelets are required for blood clotting. A drastic shortage of these blood components may lead to uncontrolled bleeding that can prove fatal.

The use of these toxic drugs to treat life-threatening disorders—leukemia, malignant lymphomas, or other forms of cancer—is justified, since the drugs are generally less dangerous than the diseases against which they are used. But rheumatoid arthritis is only rarely life-threatening. Therefore, potentially lethal drugs should be avoided. In most cases, the immunosuppressive drugs have been used only when a patient fails to respond to all other drugs and appears to be headed toward catastrophic crippling. I agree with Dr. John Lansbury of Temple University School of Medicine in Philadelphia when he states that "use of existing immunosuppressive agents might possibly be justified in older patients with advanced rheumatoid arthritis whose joints are rapidly stiffening and whose muscles are swiftly atrophying [wasting]. In all other rheumatoid arthritis patients, these drugs should be used—if at all—with the utmost restraint and caution."

In The Future—New Drugs

Almost every major pharmaceutical company in this country appears to be devising or testing a new arthritis drug. It seems to me that in the past year or two these efforts have quadrupled. So far, none of these drugs is far enough along to be ready for a rigid, well-controlled trial in the United States. While I do know of one drug that looks promising and is being tested abroad, it is too early to tell how the drug acts or what it will do. When the preliminary reports appear and there is the usual hoopla of hope and excitement, I only hope that doctors and arthritis patients will exercise sensible restraint. Remember cortisone! An instructive time table may refresh your memory:

1944—Cortisone is synthesized.

1946—Laboratory production begins but arouses little medical interest.

1948—After two years, one-half gram (one-fifty-sixth of an ounce) is made in the laboratory. Cortisone is ready for testing in man. The first patient given cortisone at the Mayo Clinic in September responds dramatically on the third day of treatment, despite being "completely crippled" by rheumatoid arthritis.

1949—The results of the treatment are made public. Because of the immediate demand, a severe cortisone shortage results. Large-scale production is begun.

1969—The National Academy of Sciences–National Research Council in a report to the Food and Drug Administration points out that the danger of treating rheumatoid diseases with steroids often outweighs the advantages of disease suppression.

From neglect, to enthusiasm, to grave caution—this was the progress of the greatest of the modern "miracle drugs." Therefore, a word to the wise—be careful before trying a new drug! Jump on no band wagon. For it may turn out to be an extremely uncomfortable, even dangerous, roller-coaster ride.

SOME GLINTS OF HOPE FROM THE SURGEON'S KNIFE

The gifted young pianist felt the first twinge in her hands while playing Bach for a rapt London audience. Two months later, she was in such pain she had to call off her concert tour. In panic, she returned home where she saw a surgeon who suggested a somewhat risky procedure, the removal of the inflamed synovial membrane surrounding the metacarpals—the five cylindrical bones between the wrist and the fingers.

The surgeon made it very clear that this operation, performed on both hands, "might make it possible" to play piano again. Like any conscientious doctor, he made it clear that the proposed surgery is not invariably successful; he could not guarantee that her rheumatoid arthritis would not recur either in her hands or in another part of the body. The young woman felt she had no option. In order to continue her promising career she had to gamble and take the chance. Luckily, she won. A month after surgery, she resumed playing.

In contrast to the case of the "lucky" pianist is another woman who worked a different set of keys—those of an office typewriter. The typist also felt severe pain, but her doctor pursued conservative medical treatment for the next year. She was doing very well until, during the fifteenth month of treatment, a flare-up of the rheumatoid arthritis led to a ruptured tendon, the whitish fiber-like cord that connects muscle to bone. An operation now was necessary. It took almost a year for normal function to return to the one hand.

In its November 10, 1967, issue, *Medical World News*, a weekly magazine for doctors, cites these two case histories because they represent the dilemma of how long to wait before surgery. But do they? Would it have been sensible to operate on the typist when her disease seemed well under control? Could the typist afford to take the time from her job and her family to risk an operation whose results no one can predict with certainty?

In this matter one collides head on with various complex value judgments that a doctor and a patient must weigh together. One must first of all admit that little in life and almost nothing in disease is clear-cut and simple. One is always confronted by alternative choices, based on estimating drawbacks versus benefits, risks versus gains. I would feel successful if all my patients and all the readers of this book were to come to terms with this concept. For it can help make them discriminate between obvious short-term benefits and slowly achieved long-term gains. It is not unlike investing in the stock market—before you plunge in you must be educated so that you understand what you are doing with your money. Do you have the means to gamble on a glamour stock that may be very risky? Or do you wish to bet on a slow but sure growth opportunity?

Dr. Robert L. Preston, clinical professor of orthopedic surgery at New York University, is one of the country's leading proponents of early synovectomy. In a recent book and in the *Medical World News* article mentioned before he presents his opinion on the value of removing the inflamed synovium as early as possible.

"There is a tendency among medical people to hope for the best," he states. "Too often they wait until the joint is completely deteriorated . . . There should be an arbitrary time limit of four months placed on the medical management of patients who show chronic inflammation of the joint and tendon sheath . . . [synovectomy should be done] without delay after the patient has been given first-class medical treatment and fails to respond. Following synovectomy, it is unusual for rheumatoid inflammation to recur regardless of the course which the systemic disease may take in other joints."

Dr. Richard H. Freyberg, an internist and emeritus clinical professor of medicine at Cornell University Medical College, disagrees. He feels that synovectomy should ideally be performed before significant irreversible damage occurs, but he sees no logic in setting a time limit "because of the wide differences in the speed of the progress of the disease and the differences in severity of the disease among patients."

"First-class medical treatment must be guided by the condition of the patient—not the calendar," he declares. "I don't want to be put in a position of having to say that six months is too early or that medical management should be carried out for a year or five years. Some patients are candidates for synovectomy early and some are never candidates for surgery."

There you have it—two top specialists disagreeing on what they consider ideal care for their patients. They agree that surgery has a place in the over-all management of rheumatoid arthritis. The question is when, how, and for whom.

This operation—and you must keep in mind this is only one of several types of surgery possible for the arthritis patient—is now being examined by a study committee of the Arthritis Foundation under the auspices of the National Center for Chronic Disease Control of the U.S. Public Health Service.

The justification for doing a synovectomy is rather simple: When rheumatoid arthritis begins, it first affects the synovial membrane and only later attacks the bone and cartilage of a joint. By removing the inflamed synovium, surgeons hope to arrest the disease process, since a new synovial membrane grows back after the diseased one has been removed. The surgical pioneers found that when they did this operation, they relieved pain significantly, and postponed the disease locally. No recurrence was seen for months and even years. When the new membrane again became inflamed, the disease did not seem quite as severe as the first time. As a consequence, the surgeons have come to believe that the earlier they do a synovectomy of the hand, knee, or other joint, the more effective it will prove.

But this remains to be shown. "Synovectomy is almost always done too late," stated Dr. Preston. It is, therefore, not as effective in preventing the progress of rheumatoid arthritis as it might be. "I would prefer to risk an occasional operation prematurely rather than doing such a high percentage too late," Dr. Preston said. But Dr. Freyberg counters this claim by pointing to his study of 100 patients whom he has seen over a period of 20 years. In more than 60 patients who had rheumatoid arthritis that affected the hands, disabling damage did not occur in the finger joints until the third year of medical treatment. Nearly 30 patients showed no damage until the tenth year of treatment. The disease took its toll slowly, he points out. While some of these patients were candidates for surgery, not all of them were. When he was at the Hospital for Special Surgery in New York, Dr. Freyberg continued to urge caution about operating, but also cooperated with surgeons on the staff in a long-range evaluation of the nature and benefits of synovectomy.

In a report presented in 1969 to the annual meeting of the American Rheumatism Association, Dr. C. S. Ranawat, as spokesman for the group that also includes surgeon Dr. Lee Ramsay Straub and Drs. José L. Granda and Marcus Rivelis, summed up their experience with 12 patients two years after they had undergone a synovectomy of the knee:

"It appears that synovectomy in properly selected patients would control the clinical manifestations of chronic inflammation in the joint for a long time, despite varying degrees of recurrence of rheumatoid inflammation. The duration of improvement would seem to depend upon the

stage of degeneration of the cartilage, activity of the rheumatoid inflammation, and response to anti-inflammatory
drug therapy."

At the same meeting, Dr. Edward S. Mongan, now of
the University of Southern California, discussed the experience with 60 patients who underwent a synovectomy
of the knee, wrist, or hand joints at the University of
Rochester Medical Center. The investigators, who included Drs. William M. Boger, Bruce C. Gilliland, and
Sanford Meyerowitz, decided to evaluate the 84 operations done on the 60 patients by assessing the following
factors: Was there pain relief? Were the joints stable?
What was the range of motion? Did a new synovium
grow? What were the changes seen on the X-ray taken
after the operation? How well did the patient function in
everyday activities? Their final ratings were expressed as
better, unchanged, and worse. After judging the status of
the joint after synovectomy, they found 43 were better,
17 unchanged, and 24 were worse. There you see the risk
involved—43 joints benefited from the operation, 41 did
not. This 50-50 risk was explained by Dr. Mongan.

"The more severe the rheumatoid arthritis, the poorer
the surgical result," he reported to his fellow rheumatologists. "Although the joint operated on was usually not
severely involved, since the synovectomies were done
chiefly for prophylactic [preventive] reasons, there was a
significant correlation between over-all severity of disease
and poor surgical results. If there were no bone erosions
before the operation, the patient did better than a patient
with erosions. Moreover, the more erosions present, the
poorer the results . . .

"All patients had physical therapy after their operation
while still in the hospital, and then were instructed to
exercise at home. Patients who had physical therapy reg-

ularly as out-patients after their operation did significantly better than those who had no formal physical
therapy after discharge from the hospital."

There were some other very interesting findings. For
instance, 59 out of 84 operated joints had regrown enough
synovial membrane so that it could be felt, about two and
a half years after the operation. This finding interestingly
complements another observation, also reported to this
1969 meeting. Regeneration of the synovium was found
to take about seven months. Evidence of this was provided by Dr. Nelson Mitchell of the Royal Victoria Hospital of Montreal. He had observed eight patients who
had undergone a knee synovectomy from two months to
five years previously.

Dr. Mitchell admitted that his report was based on a
"meager amount of evidence." He had studied the kind of
cells that regenerated in the synovial membrane and
found that the operation is justified, since diseased membranes containing those dangerous lysosomal and other
enzymes are removed. "Even if this were to be replaced
by similarly diseased tissue, it would seem to take several
months to do so, thereby resting the joint in the meantime," he pointed out.

For his group, Dr. Mongan summed up that "the older
the patient at surgery, the poorer the surgical results. The
longer the patient has had arthritis prior to surgery and
the longer they have had symptoms in the operated joint
prior to surgery, the poorer the surgical results. Patients
with more severe rheumatoid arthritis fared less well than
those with less severe disease."

Dr. Currier McEwen, professor of medicine at New
York University, is the chairman of the Arthritis Foundation's study committee that seeks within the next few
years to determine if early surgery on the synovium will

indeed prevent the disease from progressing. The committee hopes also to determine how *early* is "early." Says Dr. McEwen, "There is some evidence that if synovectomy is done early enough, it can prevent the progressive damage which is expected in the usual course of the disease. But this is still only a clinical impression, and it is not known with certainty if it is true. This study should provide the answer."

The answers should emerge from a series of studies done all over the world over the next few years. It is high time, incidentally. Synovectomy of the knee joint dates back to 1870. What has been missing since then is a clearcut "yes or no" on the usefulness of the operation. This will come only after a great number of patients who have undergone surgery have been studied for years.

"The surgeons always say it is never early enough to do a synovectomy," Dr. Bernard Rogoff, an internist at he Hospital for Special Surgery, has pointed out. "And then the orthopedic surgeons present a report six months or a year after the operation when patients are usually doing quite well. But when the treating physician continues to see these patients for five and ten years, the outlook is not so sanguine."

In my office I keep reprints of the *Medical World News* article (November 10, 1967) to show along with similar discussions of the problems of surgery to my patients in order to enlighten them about the pros and cons of referring them to a surgeon. I have always worked closely with a surgeon, and we are always debating about who is the likely candidate to be helped by surgery. Our professional discussion continues within my hospital—just as it does between orthopedic surgeons and rheumatologists throughout the country. But, to be as clear-cut as possible, here are some guidelines for patients who may be considering an operation for their rheumatoid arthritis.

OTHER SURGICAL TRUMP CARDS

There is no operation of any sort that will cure rheumatoid arthritis. Nonetheless, there are a variety of surgical procedures that must be considered as part of the individualized treatment plan for the rheumatoid patient.

There are types of surgery that are preventive, such as the previously discussed "early" synovectomies. Other types of surgery seek to repair or salvage a joint that is severely affected or even deformed. Whatever the procedure thought suitable, it is used to help alleviate a patient's pain, to improve the function of a joint, or to correct an already existing crippling deformity. Among the procedures, the following are the most frequent:

For the hip, arthroplasty—any surgical repair of the bone—will help to relieve pain. There are various kinds. In far-advanced problems, total replacement of the hip joint is the newest technique. The bones that form the hip, the femoral head and the acetabulum, are replaced by artificial components that are cemented into place. To bond the metal implant to the bone, a plastic substance, an acrylic, is used. The discovery of this bonding technique is considered the great milestone in total replacement arthroplasty, which is now the "operation of choice" for many surgeons.

For the knee, various procedures are available: synovectomy; joint debridement—literally the cleaning up or removal of all foreign matter or inflamed or dead tissue; arthrodesis, in which a joint is fixed or fused so that it becomes immobile; osteotomy, where a bone is surgically cut above or below the joint to permit the correction of a deformity.

For the spine and neck, fusion of the vertebrae high in the spine (at a location of the cervical spine called C-1 and C-2) has been performed when an X-ray reveals a subluxation, a partial dislocation. The surgery will not only fix the dislocation, but, importantly, will prevent pinching of the nerve.

For the foot, removal of the heads of the metatarsal bones, the five long bones between the toes and the tarsus (the bones of the ankle and heel) as well as removal of part of the toe bones will afford relief.

For the hand, many of these procedures are used—synovectomy, joint debridement, arthrodesis, or arthroplasty; sometimes these procedures are combined with the replacement and reworking of injured tendons. There are at least four different types of artificial finger joints currently in use, including metal-hinge joints and those made of a synthetic material.

Because the hand is like the face, constantly exposed and used, surgeons have concentrated on ways to preserve its function. Repair and salvage procedures have become increasingly sophisticated, and rightly so. One cannot describe the tremendous value of surgery, both physically and psychologically, when a previously deformed hand—one that could not hold or grasp anything, that seemed to have lost all strength—is suddenly able to perform almost as well as before the rheumatoid arthritis struck. Some surgeons have described the dismay of rheumatoid patients when, delighted with the result of one surgical procedure, they contemplate what else has to be done. It has been my experience that once surgery has succeeded, patients seem willing to undergo any number of subsequent operations. Some of my patients have been incredibly courageous in the face of what I consider endless surgery.

An example of this was Elizabeth Fentell, who had advanced rheumatoid arthritis that affected almost all her joints. She was unable to walk because of her painful hips and she could not use crutches, since her hand and elbow were painfully swollen and restricted in movement. Although past 50, she was undaunted when surgery was first performed on her hand, and then on her elbow, in order to allow her to use crutches. Then a knee and both hips were operated on. Today, about three years after these series of operations were begun, she walks with the use of a cane. It was her admirable courage that allowed her to walk where once she was mostly confined to bed.

The example of Elizabeth Fentell also shows the approach an orthopedic surgeon and I use with a patient. That is, as part of the team in the hospital, we will plot the sequence of surgical procedures. When a patient has disability of both the arms and hands and also of the legs and hips, then we will start on the hands and arms before tackling the problems of the legs. This is done because of the general agreement among surgeons and physicians that it is far more important, physically and psychologically, to ease the difficulties of eating, dressing, or other matters of personal care—most of my patients complain especially about the difficulties they have combing their hair. So it is easy to understand why surgery of the hands, wrists, or elbows takes precedence.

A major consideration before undertaking any surgery is the condition of a rheumatoid patient. Surgery is not done on a patient during a flare-up of disease; we wait until an attack subsides. Surgeons are also extremely reluctant to operate on the bed-ridden patient, unless, as in the case of Elizabeth Fentell, confinement to bed has been only for a matter of a few months. Those bed-ridden for years are considered poor "operative risks," because it is generally thought that they will recuperate very slowly and painfully after an operation, and that some tissues may possibly not heal at all.

The willingness of both patients and doctors to consider surgery has been one of the most encouraging developments of recent years. It would have been unthinkable as little as ten years ago to undergo the number of operations some rheumatoid patients have permitted. But then, who would have thought a decade ago that a patient would allow a surgeon to remove a diseased heart and have it replaced by a donor's healthy heart? Of course, some people would never consider such an extreme measure, although, it appears, there are few ungrateful heart transplant patients—even when life has been lengthened by only a relatively short span.

For the arthritis patient, there is less urgency than for the heart patient. Yet, the rheumatologist is like the heart specialist, the cardiologist. He prefers to treat his patients with all the medical means at his command before he suggests surgery.

The measures discussed up to this point should, under ordinary conditions, prevent the extreme twisting, bending, or contraction of the joints, as well as the muscle shrinking or atrophy seen in far-advanced rheumatoid arthritis. Fortunately, the plastic or orthopedic surgeons —the latter specializes more in problems of muscles and bones—have long been comrades and partners of the physicians specializing in the treatment of arthritics. Today, surgeons are being consulted far more early in treatment than in former days. Also, surgeons frequently see an arthritis patient before a rheumatologist does, and have become more proficient in treating the rheumatoid patient by *medical* means. For in the last analysis, surgery is the trump card played late in the game—not always, but usually. It is wise, therefore, to hold the winning cards until one is ready to play them. For the chance always exists that you may not win. Among the major advances must be counted the number of surgical procedures available today. If one does not achieve the desired goal at first, one may try again, cautiously, of course.

I don't wish to push the similarity between the game of cards and the treatment of the rheumatoid patient. Yet, a physician tries to play each card tellingly in favor of his patient. This may engender great arguments—such as those between the surgeons and the internists about the value of surgery. These discussions are in behalf of the best of possible care, and the more vociferous, the better. Patients and doctors will surely benefit as long as the professionals lay their cards on the table and openly discuss the pros and cons of a technique that seeks to improve the lot of their patients.

NONMEDICAL ASSISTANCE TO RHEUMATOID PATIENTS

I have been increasingly concerned over the years to help my patients in problems that are not strictly medical, but that influence the progress they are likely to make in combatting a disease as difficult and treacherous, as complex and anxiety-provoking, as rheumatoid arthritis. It is my obligation to refer a patient to a surgeon or to a psychiatrist if I feel it necessary. Similarly, I also have a social obligation in trying to help settle financial, family, job, or sexual problems. Since I have spent my entire professional life in large university-connected hospitals, this has been a relatively simple matter. Social workers have been an integral part of the treatment team, and they have worked with patients who needed guidance about changing jobs, finding part-time help to take care of the house, especially during a period of active disease, and even with helping to find ways to finance long-term medical care.

Most often the hospital social worker can aid a patient in getting in touch with a vocational rehabilitation specialist who will help find a training or a new job, if the present one is too strenuous or taxing. But a patient can also help himself. A list of rehabilitation services can be obtained by getting a copy of "Medicine's Back to Work Plan" from the American Medical Association Committee on Rehabilitation (535 N. Dearborn, Chicago, Ill. 60610) or from the National Rehabilitation Association (1522 K Street, N.W., Washington, D.C. 20005).

The need for spreading knowledge about rehabilitation services, whether medical or vocational, is obviously very great. In the spring of 1969, Mary E. Switzer, the Federal Social and Rehabilitation Administrator, noted that one-fourth of all disabled persons interviewed in a survey had not received rehabilitation services, nor did they know where to seek such help.

Moreover, among all the households surveyed, few knew how or where to get aid, suggesting the Federal Government or telephone operators as sources of rehabilitation services. "The survey confirmed our long-held suspicions," Miss Switzer stated, "that the availability of help for the disabled is, unfortunately, still largely unknown. Yet, over 200,000 disabled persons were restored to productive lives [in 1968]. It is estimated that there are at least five million disabled Americans who may be eligible for rehabilitation services."

Among the disabilities included were those due to blindness, mental retardation, or crippling due to a birth defect. However, the same applies to the rheumatoid arthritis patient. More of these patients need to learn where to seek help in trying to obtain special therapy for a specific physical problem and/or to take advantage of available vocational training.

MAY BARTON'S PROGRESS

Despite having the same severe disease that Marlene Smith had, May Barton made a remarkable recovery. And that lengthy first day of instruction proved instrumental in helping May Barton to begin her treatment. On the first day, she may not have understood everything that she learned. But she did walk home that evening with the knowledge that a great deal could and would be done for her. And she knew that whatever the question, she could get an answer either from the treatment team at the clinic or from one of the many booklets and pamphlets she had been given that day.

Most important, May Barton learned that she and the team were partners, that we would work together to achieve the most important goal in the life of a rheumatoid arthritis patient—the continuation of as normal a life as possible. She also knew that whatever the progress of her disease, she would get complete and thorough support from us. This in itself helped. When I next saw May, she admitted that she had arrived home totally exhausted, but so happy and relieved that she slept well and easily that night, and did not mind the pain.

The specific treatment provided May proved to be remarkably simple; fortunately, she believed in it as being suited to her needs. She began by taking aspirin—up to 20 five-grain tablets every day. She developed ringing in the ears which disappeared after she took two fewer aspirins daily. Soon, her joints were less painful and warm, and she could move them more readily. This permitted her to start physical therapy and exercises. She took a hot tub bath every morning to ease the morning stiffness; she dipped both hands in hot paraffin. After the bath and the heat treatment she would exercise, just as she had been taught at the clinic. Soon, there was increasing motion in the knees, wrists, and hands.

At the beginning of treatment, when her wrists and hands were hot and tender due to the rheumatoid inflammation, she wore resting splints at night. These had been prepared for her at the clinic so that she should not bend her wrists but keep them straight. Without these splints, May would have developed a flexion deformity of the wrist—which she would hold bent to ease the discomfort. This deformity might have developed within a matter of weeks, but the splints prevented it.

At first, we saw May every week. She found that by taking one or more short rest periods every day, she could avoid the terribly overwhelming fatigue she had felt early in mid-afternoon. We had originally suggested only one short rest period during the day, but she found that a second rest of about half an hour was necessary. During the early phases of treatment, we made several readjustments in May's treatment program. We changed the amount of aspirin and the type of exercises she was doing. Within a year our efforts had borne fruit. May was back at work as a secretary, had little discomfort, and no disability.

After three years, May Barton, in contrast with Marlene Smith, was doing very nicely. She is still taking aspirin, 15 tablets a day, but she is also receiving gold injections once a month. She never needed steroids, fortunately, and she is sanguine about the future—feeling that she will maintain her present gains in the future.

Interestingly enough, it was May who supplied me with a list of don'ts that she had found valuable. Here are May's general precautions on what not to do during her day-to-day activities, her "remember to avoid" list:

• Don't hold any joint or muscle too long in one position. This will impede circulation and put pressure on one side of a joint instead of distributing the pressure equally.

• Don't do any sustained physical activity without a short interruption for a rest period.

• Don't sit for more than thirty minutes without moving. It may help to elevate and pad the chair with pillows. Don't "flop down" into a chair, instead lower yourself gently. When getting up, don't push against a table, gently use the sides of the chair to help you stand up.

• Don't pull an object, always push, using your leg muscles rather than straining your arms. Use the knees instead of the back while lifting an object. Don't push against the fingers, use the palms.

• Don't lift heavy objects, such as a roasting pan, by the handle. Use a glove-type pot holder, and lift from the bottom.

• Don't use tools with small grip-type handles. Convert them to larger handles or purchase specially prepared tools with large, wide grips.

• Don't ever slouch, walk straight and erect.

• Don't do anything that puts too much force against the fingers, such as forcing a drawer open. This may seriously injure a vulnerable joint.

• Don't sleep with pillows under your neck or knees if

either is affected by rheumatoid arthritis. This will promote flexion deformities and disability. Don't have bed sheets or blankets drawn tightly over your feet.

• Don't do routine things that somehow tend to promote discomfort or deformity, such as clutching a purse by the fingers; carry the purse on the arm near the elbow. Above all, don't use daily activities as part of the exercise program. Instead, simplify the housework to make time available for heat treatments and exercise. They have priority.

• Don't be misled into thinking that you can do your household chores as easily and quickly as your friends and neighbors. Do adjust your life to this fact of your existence.

• Don't feel it is wrong for you to have some domestic help, help with the laundry, nursery school for younger children, as many gadgets as possible in the kitchen. Perhaps you should redesign the kitchen to make it as comfortable for you as possible.

• Don't ever hesitate to turn to your physician with a problem. You may have accepted the fact that there is no cure for rheumatoid arthritis, but he may suggest something else that might be done to help, even when you feel that nothing more can really be done.

• Don't despair. Remember that research is pushing ahead at unprecedented rates in the field of arthritis. Perhaps soon, transplantation of joints will be a reality!

It is from these large and small do's and don'ts that May Barton and untold rheumatoid arthritis patients like her have constructed useful and relatively undisturbed lives. The current state of care for the rheumatoid patient is encouraging, far happier than it was even a few years ago. Perhaps most comforting will be the day, soon at hand, when the words rheumatoid arthritis no longer in-spire fear and terror or the image of a helplessly crippled relative or friend. Rather the image of May Barton will be the standard, the typical rheumatoid patient, who is both well informed and doing well.

III. *Children with Rheumatoid Arthritis*

> Humanity has but three great enemies: fever, famine, and war; of these by far the greatest, by far the most terrible, is fever.
>
> SIR WILLIAM OSLER

EVERY PARENT will readily agree with Dr. Osler's appraisal of fever as one of humanity's great enemies. You know the worry caused by a baby's high temperature, and it often seems as if a child's life is a long procession of fevers. You are scared, when the thermometer suddenly reads 105 degrees or more, which you know is dangerously high for an adult, although it is not unusual in a child. It is fortunate, then, that most often childhood fevers are not symptomatic of anything much more serious than that popular grab-bag of vague ailments—your doctor says your child has a cold, the flu, or a virus.

But no fever should be neglected or lightly dismissed. For once in a while, a high temperature does indicate something is seriously wrong. It was just such a fever that prompted my first interest in arthritis and led to my specializing in the care and treatment of children with rheumatoid arthritis.

People are usually astounded to learn that children develop rheumatoid arthritis. And so was I. About twenty years ago when I was still a medical student at Georgetown University Medical Center, I became concerned about Donna Rafferty, a bright and charming seven-year-old. Her fever—often above 105 degrees—had lasted for weeks, and appeared and vanished sometimes as often as twice a day. Donna's knees were warm and swollen to the point where she could barely move them. Furthermore, I was shocked to notice that her hands, wrists, and elbows already appeared somewhat deformed. It was obvious also that she was not growing normally. And no one could explain those fever spikes. For days on end Donna would suddenly have enormously high fever, and a few hours later would be completely fever-free, yet she did not seem very sick or even unwell. It was as if she were untouched by her high temperatures.

I did not know then that I was observing one of the telltale symptoms of the acute form of juvenile rheumatoid arthritis. The cause for the fever remains a mystery. Later I was to discover that this mysterious waxing and waning fever is very often accompanied by a skin eruption that usually appears and disappears with the fever. Juvenile rheumatoid arthritis is obviously a disease that attacks the entire body, not just the joints. But I am getting ahead of my story. This was twenty years ago, Donna Rafferty was the first child I had ever seen that had arthritis, and I still remember how appalled and heartsick I was that Donna's doctors and all my teachers thought that very little could be done to keep Donna from becoming completely crippled. Perhaps the newly discovered cortisone might be useful, they said. Of course, as you learned in the chapter on adults with rheumatoid arthritis, cortisone is usually the worst possible drug to use first, and certainly cannot be used for a long period of time. In children, cortisone-type drugs are particularly hazardous because they will stunt normal growth.

Donna was a child with a strange and worrisome malady. During the previous three years, she had been in the hospital four times. But none of the doctors could decide what was the matter. She had had "fever of unknown origin." Now that the doctors knew what Donna's illness was, they were little better equipped to help her, since there was so little definitive knowledge about her disease. They continued to be in a quandary about what to do, and were ready to try anything new that might help. And that is why cortisone was tried. It was a tragic mistake.

For Donna died. It took two years, and she died not from her arthritis, but from the then unknown and unsuspected complications of cortisone therapy. Earlier I cited the story of another little girl who suffered a similar fate many years later. But you must understand that in Donna's case, the intentions were the best. Today, unless no other drug can help, the internal use of cortisone or similar drugs in the treatment of children with rheumatoid arthritis should be avoided. One of my major efforts has been to educate the medical profession about the potential harm that these drugs can do when they are given to children. There is no reason for them to be given unless no other drug will work or a specific complication of the disease requires the use of a cortisone-type of drug.

Keep in mind that I am now talking about the cortisone children take internally. Cortisone injected directly into a joint is quite another matter. This is an extremely useful procedure, and you need have few qualms about it. It should not be done too frequently. But when it is performed, it usually proves quite effective in reducing pain and improving the capacity to move.

All this I was to learn only later, after I had determined to begin a thorough study of all aspects of juvenile rheumatoid arthritis.

In Washington, D.C., Donna Rafferty had not been my patient. Neither was the little girl in California. But both little girls, one nine, one 13, when they died, have had a profound influence on my professional life.

Such tragedies make me both sad and indignant. Too often at fault are doctors or parents who do not know enough. Twenty years ago, when I consulted all the experts I could find to talk to and when I read all the available medical literature, the outlook for children with rheumatoid arthritis was bleak. A simple, pessimistic formula stated what doctors then believed: One-third of the children supposedly died, one-third were doomed to become severely deformed, and the remaining third were sure to content with all manner of physical difficulties throughout their life. Juvenile rheumatoid arthritis was a hideous, life-long affliction.

That was what the doctors believed in 1950. But today, in the 1970s, the outlook for children with rheumatoid arthritis is enormously brighter, although the disease remains what it has always been, potentially the major chronic, progressive crippler of children, a long-term malady that affects perhaps a quarter of a million youngsters in the United States. You will be shocked to learn, as I was, that some victims of rheumatoid arthritis are still in their earliest infancy. My youngest patient was only six weeks old. I have treated a number of infants who were only a few months old. Most children I treat are from one to three years old. I see twice as many girls as boys.

For the past two decades I have seen hundreds of children with juvenile rheumatoid arthritis. I have studied them, and for as long as possible have followed their progress. It has taken a lot of time, and it has been a painstaking process. But it has been a source of enormous satisfaction to me to be contributing to the knowledge about juvenile rheumatoid arthritis that has been accumulating in this country and abroad. Fortunately, more and more arthritis specialists are particularly interested in children.

For parents, perhaps the most important new knowledge is simply this: There are really three kinds of juvenile rheumatoid arthritis—each is quite different in the way it begins, continues, and should be treated. All three forms are quite different from the adult disease and from other childhood arthritic conditions—rheumatic fever, traumatic, tuberculous, or infectious arthritis. For you the most significant advance today is the ever greater assurance that a great deal can be done for a child with rheumatoid arthritis. And there is less and less chance for a child to die or be crippled.

By now I have been involved in the treatment of hundreds of children. And as I continue to see more and more children, I become increasingly more hopeful about their outlook for the future.

My enthusiasm for what we can now do for a child with rheumatoid arthritis derives from the more than 300 children whom I have been studying from the day they first came to see me. (I have seen many others as a consultant.) A few are now over 25; many have been my patients for up to 15 years. A group of 100—they are from 10 to 28 years old—so I hesitate to call them children— have been treated by me continuously for 10 years or more. And what have I learned from them? Since so little was known, everything had to be studied. What is juvenile rheumatoid arthritis really like? How does it begin?

Very high fever and rash that comes and goes, and is

accompanied by some discomfort, but by little or no puffiness of the joints—these are the first signs of acute juvenile rheumatoid arthritis. One three-year-old girl was to have these symptoms for fully nine years. It was not until she was 12 years old that the first objective signs of arthritis, that is, swelling or puffiness of a joint, were observed. Up to then, the little girl had complained of some pain in the joints, arthralgia, as it is called. This is admittedly an unusual example of acute beginning disease. Only one out of every five children with juvenile rheumatoid arthritis is likely to have an acute form of disease. These children have the dramatic symptoms, but are likely to appear in reasonably good health.

Half of the children with juvenile rheumatoid arthritis begin with a polyarticular onset—more than four joints are affected, are painful, stiff, and swollen, but there is only some fever or rash. Such children look ill, they are listless, refuse to eat, and are losing weight. Often, this form begins "silently," and the only way you can tell your child is having joint pain is by the curious way he or she lies in bed; the child does not move around as much as before, or lies with his knees flexed. There is tenderness of the joints, rather than pain. Also, a child may limp a little, but does not complain of pain. These are early signals that the disease may be beginning.

These two forms account for almost three-quarters of the kinds of juvenile rheumatoid arthritis one is likely to see. Two out of ten children will have acute disease at the beginning (few or no swollen joints), five of ten have polyarticular disease (more than four joints affected), and three of ten have monarticular juvenile rheumatoid arthritis (swelling of only one joint—most often the knee —for a minimum of one month). Children with monarticular beginning disease appear in good health, other than their complaint about the painful knee. Only if they are under the age of five are they likely to have fever, appear ill, listless, and irritable.

You must remember that these three beginnings are like the tips of icebergs—the great preponderance of what the disease will be like is hidden from view. But what does the future hold for these children?

Let me give you some examples. This is what happened to Keith Kerr during the ten years of my treatment.

HIGH FEVER PLUS RASH PLUS JOINT PAIN SUGGESTS ACUTE DISEASE

Keith was six months old when he first began to have high fever, rash, and joint pain. His first attack—and each of 40 subsequent ones—lasted only two weeks. During the second week of his first attack, his parents became so worried that they took him to a hospital. But after a week the Kerrs took their son home without ever knowing what he had. The doctors had told them little, other than that Keith's spleen was enlarged, as were most of the lymph glands of his body, particularly the ones under the arms and in the neck.

I did not see Keith until he was six years old. By that time, as I mentioned, he had experienced 41 attacks of fever and rash—they would appear every six weeks to four months; there was nothing too regular about their appearance. During the years of these attacks, Keith had perhaps felt a twinge of discomfort in an elbow, knee, or other joint, but aside from occasional swelling, no real disability. There was little indication, therefore, that this child might have arthritis. He was well when I saw him—in between his attacks—and nothing could be found, either by examination or X-ray, that would suggest joint involvement. Only my experience with other children led me to conclude that this little boy was suffering from recurrent short-lived attacks of juvenile rheumatoid arthritis—a form of the disease I call polycyclic (many cycles) acute febrile (fever) disease.

Once I decided what was wrong, I put Keith on aspirin whenever he had an attack. It was all he really needed during the week or two that his attacks would last. The amount of aspirin was adjusted to his body weight, so that he received up to one grain per pound daily. Keith weighed 62 pounds and had to take 10 baby aspirin tablets (1¼ grain) five times a day. This is a lot of aspirin, but smaller quantities, those you might use for slight or low-grade fevers, are just not effective to control these episodes of high fever. Eventually, Keith took 12 adult five-grain tablets each day, once he had learned to swallow them.

It was the diligent keeping of daily fever records by Mrs. Kerr that helped me to establish the correct diagnosis. She found that fever spikes occurred once or twice daily, going as high as 105 or 106 degrees. Temperature then fell to 98.6 and even subnormal levels of 96 to 97 degrees. The wide variation of temperatures, from the very low of 96 to a high of 106, with one to two peaks daily, is typical of childhood rheumatoid arthritis.

The prominence of high fever in children, unlike adults with rheumatoid arthritis, was first described in 1896 by Dr. George F. Still at London's Great Ormond Street Hospital for Sick Children (where I was later to receive some of my training). But no one paid attention to the relationship between fever and juvenile rheumatoid arthritis until Professor E. G. L. Bywaters, one of my teachers at the Postgraduate Medical School of London, made the connection more than fifty years later.

Observation of the typical fever alone is not sufficient to make a diagnosis of juvenile rheumatoid arthritis. Other disease manifestations provide important clues in establishing a definitive diagnosis. These include enlargement of the spleen, liver, or lymph glands, pericarditis, an inflammation of the lining sac of the heart, and, most important of all, a characteristic rash that is present in practically all patients whose disease begins with high fever.

What makes the rash of juvenile rheumatoid arthritis different from those that accompany measles, rubella, or chicken pox?

The characteristic rash rarely itches like the skin eruptions found in measles and similar childhood disorders. The rash may come and go, usually as the fever rises and falls, and keeps recurring for months and years. This is what makes this skin eruption very different from those short-lived rashes of measles or other childhood diseases.

Rash occurs in almost half the children with rheumatoid arthritis. But it is present in about 90 percent of all cases of acute febrile onset. Like fever, therefore, it provides the physician with clues to an early diagnosis of the acute disease at a time when very little else suggests an arthritic condition.

Fever and rash are not usually present at the time I examine a patient. The parents merely report that they observed fever and rash. In such instances, I stroke or gently scratch the upper abdomen with my fingers. If, after a couple of minutes, a telltale rash appears over the scratchmarks, I am well on my way to a definite diagnosis. Any parent can do this and elicit this manifestation, which is known as the Koebner phenomenon—chains of isolated red blotches (macules) are triggered by gentle stroking. A brighter, more florid rash occurs due to pressure of bedsheets or where the skin is rubbed or irritated by tight clothing.

The rash you see might be confused with other skin eruptions. But blotches due to juvenile rheumatoid arthritis are relatively small in size and tend to appear on the face, palms, and soles; these places are rarely the sites of other rashes, such as the one seen in rheumatic fever. Remember, there are few rashes of childhood disorders that are as highly evanescent, or recur as regularly with fever spikes, as does the rash of juvenile rheumatoid arthritis.

What happens to Keith and children who begin with an acute mode of onset? One out of two eventually develops arthritis, sometimes within the first year but occasionally as long as nine to ten years after having had multiple acute attacks.

The other patient continues to have recurrent attacks of fever and rash and joint pain, sometimes even swelling of joints. Attacks vary in frequency from only one to as many as ten in a single year. Eventually, acute attacks stop. Keith is now 16 and has been well for two years. But during the years of his polycyclic acute febrile disease, he had well over one hundred attacks of fever.

PAINFUL HAND, FOOT, KNEE, AND WRIST EQUALS POLYARTICULAR DISEASE

Frank Benton began to have pain and swelling in many joints when he was nine. Within a year, he had developed swelling of the knuckles and fingers, the joints of the foot, and the knees, wrists, and elbows.

After a year of treatment with aspirin, supportive splints, and exercises, there was no evidence of joint swelling anywhere. It was as if his disease had stopped.

This happens frequently; during the second year of disease, a temporary remission may occur spontaneously.

Three years later, shortly after a routine check-up, Frank again began to have pain and swelling of both knees, ankles, and particularly the heels. He had to come in almost weekly for check-ups, sometimes for injections of his tender heels.

Frank had to contend with an unusual home situation. His mother, an obnoxious woman, always threatened to take her son to other doctors; she had taken Frank to many doctors before she first brought him to me. Nothing satisfied her. It was Frank who made the decision to come and see me although he was only 13 at the time. He never told his mother. He would see me after school for treatments, with his father's approval, and was adamant in refusing to see any other doctor his mother suggested.

Frank is now 18 and finishing high school; fortunately he has no further trouble with his arthritis.

PROBLEMS OF DIAGNOSIS

Your doctor may hesitate in diagnosing your child's early polyarticular juvenile rheumatoid arthritis. He may want to see if the swelling of the joints lasts for more than a month or two. If so, it is juvenile rheumatoid arthritis, and the possibility of rheumatic fever or of an untoward reaction to a drug or vaccine has been ruled out. Only a short-lived arthritis is observed in these conditions.

You may have heard about a recent newcomer among vaccine reactions. This is the arthritis that small children sometimes get after they have received their shot against German measles (rubella). You can consider this a "disease of medical progress." It appears in a few days and sometimes even up to six weeks after immunization. But this side effect will soon disappear spontaneously; at the longest it might take a month and a half. During this time, a little aspirin will serve to make a child a good deal more comfortable.

RHEUMATIC FEVER

Juvenile rheumatoid arthritis is most often confused with rheumatic fever. This is a serious inflammatory disease that occurs after a "strep throat" (specifically, an infection of group A streptococcus). Although the word "rheumatic" in the name emphasizes the arthritis observed in this disease, the importance of rheumatic fever lies in the damage it may cause to a child's heart. The disease may prove fatal during its acute phase, or it can cause chronic scarring or deformity of the heart valves.

The arthritis of rheumatic fever is not really too important. What matters is that the disease merely "licks at the joints, but *bites* at the heart," according to an old saying. Rheumatic fever is no longer the threat it once was. Doctors report seeing much less of the disease; this is also my experience. Years ago in New Jersey, I remember seeing about a hundred cases during a spring epidemic of strep sore throats. But during three years in California, I saw only one case.

Some specialists now believe that one of the greatest advances in the field of rheumatology during the past twenty years has been this "near disappearance" of rheumatic fever. The widespread use of penicillin and other antibiotics, together with a natural waning of the amount and virulence of the group A streptococci, may have influenced the decline of strep epidemics. Generally improved public health and social conditions, as well as the great alertness mothers show about taking care of their children's sore throats, may also have contributed to the decrease of rheumatic fever. Children are still getting it, but it is less likely to cause permanent heart disease. Recent research has been reassuring in this matter, since it has shown that the child who does not develop heart disease as part of the first acute phase of rheumatic fever will escape the injury caused by later attacks. Only the child who has already sustained heart valve damage is at risk of more harm from subsequent attacks. These are the only children who must receive monthly shots of penicillin as a preventive measure against subsequent infection with group A streptococci. A vaccine against streptococci is a soon-to-be-fulfilled promise. Hopefully, it will prove as effective as other types of immunization. Then rheumatic fever may really be completely conquered and will assume only historic interest as a form of childhood arthritis.

THE FLOWER GIRL WITH MONARTICULAR DISEASE

When I first saw Laura Adriani, I had no idea she would be the flower girl at my wedding. How could I have known that the tearful little girl who limped because her knees were swollen, painful, and stiff would precede my bride-to-be down the aisle? But eventually there was Laura, sprinkling rose petals as she went, causing everyone present to exclaim how adorable she looked! And she practically waltzed up the aisle during the wedding march.

Laura was only two when she developed arthritis in her right knee. It happened so subtly that her parents did not notice, and Laura never complained. But eventually the parents saw that their little girl limped slightly when she was overtired. After a while, Laura developed swelling of the opposite knee, a low-grade fever, and some slight anemia. Her parents and, particularly her grandmother, all of whom are involved in the running of one of New York's finest restaurants, became tremendously upset to see signs of early crippling. Laura limped and cried out in pain, and her family was in despair.

She was sent to me by the late great rheumatologist, Dr. Russell Cecil, who knew of my special interest in children. I shall not soon forget that visit. It took four hours to conduct the examination, including the X-rays and laboratory tests, and to learn all about Laura's medical history, and then to explain what Laura's form of the disease really was. I remember her father had tears in his eyes when he learned that his little girl would probably not be crippled for life, as he had feared. And, like most parents, he was amazed at how simple the treatment turned out to be!

"Management," as the fancy medical phrase goes, consisted of giving Laura 10 grains of aspirin five times a day. Her mother applied heat packs to each knee for 20 minutes twice a day, and then Laura and her father or mother did some specially prescribed knee exercises. Occasionally, during the first month, I removed some of the fluid from the knee and would also inject a corticosteroid medication. I was seeing Laura every two weeks at the arthritis clinic. Nothing dramatic, nothing drastic was done, but within three months, the knees no longer hurt because the swelling had disappeared.

During the years since then, Laura has had two brief recurrences of her disease. Each time one knee became swollen; in both instances she had fallen or injured her knee. The same conservative measures were used—some aspirin, some heat treatment, some exercises. I also removed some fluid from the knee with a syringe—and then injected a corticosteroid solution to ease the pain and inflammation. This is all it took to control Laura's disease.

Vigilance about an unusual complication—the possible loss of vision due to cataracts—must be kept up in patients such as Laura. Every three months she must be checked to be sure that she has no early signs of a serious eye problem called chronic iridocyclitis. This inflammation of the anterior chamber of the eye comes on suddenly and without any warning symptoms, so that only a slit lamp examination by an eye specialist, an ophthalmologist, can help prevent blindness due to this dangerous complication. All children with juvenile rheumatoid arthritis are likely to develop this condition and therefore should have this simple and painless examination done every six months. But most susceptible are the children who have the monarticular beginning disease and who have the least arthritis subsequently; they need to be examined every three months.

Today, ten years after Laura's disease was first diagnosed, a slit lamp examination every three months has become routine. Such watchful prevention is all the "treatment" she receives.

Laura has continued to grow normally and has now developed into a beautiful preadolescent. It is as if the days when she limped and was in pain are completely forgotten. Even though she cannot be considered absolutely cured, she does not have any sort of symptom that would indicate that she has chronic and perhaps life-long disease. And although she has had two recurrences of her disease with one knee painfully swollen, the likelihood is very good that she may eventually "outgrow" her juvenile rheumatoid arthritis, although there is no absolute assurance of this. Her parents are aware that for many years to come Laura will have to have regular check-ups at the arthritis clinic. But for now every six months is enough. Four visits to the ophthalmologist and two visits to the arthritis clinic every year are all that Laura needs.

For children as well as for adults with rheumatoid arthritis, simple measures can often achieve remarkable results! Because so many people are so conditioned to new and marvelous miracle drugs or surgical feats, it is difficult for them to accept the simple means. And, unfortunately, many doctors really don't understand the different types of juvenile rheumatoid arthritis or they give in to parental expectations by treating dramatic symptoms with drastic medications. In juvenile rheumatoid arthritis, such an approach may be as damaging as the disease itself.

In Laura's case, there had been much head scratching and puzzlement. Her first doctors could not believe that her arthritis would be confined to only the knees. They suspected that Laura would ultimately have arthritis in many joints. It was this frightening prospect—the likelihood that Laura would have increasing pain and disability—that caused the family to become despondent about the future. Laura's grandmother even confessed to me that she had for a wild moment considered taking the sick little girl in her arms and jumping off a nearby bridge. Such excessive emotions are understandable. There is little in life worse than having to watch a young child suffer without being able to help.

But because I was able to help, Laura's family has ever since treated me as if I were some sort of marvelous magician. I have received the credit for averting what would *not* have happened in any case, and nothing I could do to explain this has kept Laura's grandmother from treating me as if I were the fabled Houdini who had pulled off a masterful escape act. As it turned out, it was Laura's grandmother who actually provided some magic.

For she soon discovered that we were neighbors in New York, and that I was a bachelor who often ate out. It became a matter of pride and principle for Laura's grandmother that I had to eat at her wonderful restaurant, and to this day I have never been allowed to pick up a check. But that was not enough. She went on to arrange a blind date for me one Sunday night. Months later I married the girl. At the wedding, Laura attracted more attention than the bride. And she keeps on being the cutest member of a wedding. I recently received a new photograph—Laura, now 12, all pink and white and adorable in her flower girl's outfit.

NEW HOPE FOR THE CHILD WITH RHEUMATOID ARTHRITIS

The children I have been discussing have all been helped. So far, I have found that, for nine out of ten children, the long-term outlook is excellent. This is a far cry from only twenty years ago, when most arthritis specialists believed that juvenile rheumatoid arthritis was untreatable, could not be halted, and would maim or kill its victims.

Today, pessimism has given way to a far more realistic and hopeful approach. Today there is no excuse to delay or avoid treatment. In fact, the sooner a child begins treatment, the better will be the results. I have found that children who were treated during the first year of their disease have achieved more than those whom I saw two to four years or more after they became ill.

Treatment of juvenile rheumatoid arthritis has really

only one, very logical aim: A childhood and adolescence as normal and undisturbed as possible. It is a pleasure to report that this aim can be achieved for most children. Juvenile rheumatoid arthritis can be treated successfully by simple, uncomplicated, conservative means. Home care is the cornerstone of treatment, and this means heat application and exercising. As for drugs, aspirin is all that was needed in 89 of the 100 children, all of whom I have treated now for 10 years or more; as yet, only three children have received oral cortisone-like drugs for more than one year, and only eight are receiving gold injections. Since 60 of the 100 children have no disease and are receiving no treatment, you can see why I have become increasingly enthusiastic about simple, conservative management.

What about the other 40 children? Twenty-nine continue to be treated conservatively and are doing very well, although they have active disease. Nine children have done poorly. They have not grown normally and they are contending with various physical problems; their movements are constricted, and they have trouble turning their heads; their childhood is not normal. They are the testimony to the appalling fact that juvenile rheumatoid arthritis is a serious, potentially crippling disease.

In this tally, two children remain. And, sad to say, they died. One was a beautiful little girl who began to have acute disease with fever and rash when she was two years old. A year later, a rare and dreadful complication of the disease was discovered. This is amyloidosis, the formation of a white, crystalline substance that settles between the cells of the body structure. Once the kidney is infiltrated by amyloid, it stops functioning normally, and life is threatened. Amyloidosis as a disease is just beginning to be understood, but as yet there is nothing that can be done to prevent its lethal effects. The little girl died five years later, when she was eight.

Her death is the only one that was due to rheumatoid arthritis. The other patient, 19 years old, died because of an overwhelming infection he developed after he underwent surgery for a crippled knee. So the disease was only indirectly responsible. Both were among the 11 patients whose disease went progressively downhill, despite the most vigorous attempts by the team of doctors, surgeons, and rehabilitation specialists that I headed at the Jersey City Medical Center juvenile arthritis clinic.

In my experience, only one child out of ten, rather than two out of three as in former times, becomes physically handicapped by severe deformities. These children suffer from constant and progressive flexion deformities, so that they cannot completely extend their arms and legs. Three of these patients are confined to wheelchairs. Severe deformities are most often the result of progressive arthritis of the hips and knees.

As for the fatalities, it may seem callous to cite statistics. Yet there is a great difference when I think of the prediction of death for one out of every three children and compare it with my sufficiently disheartening experience of two deaths among 100 patients.

All this juggling of figures is meaningless in terms of human suffering. But the figures do indicate that great progress has been made in juvenile rheumatoid arthritis. There is more cause for optimism about the treatment of this disease than ever before. The only area where little or no progress has been made is in the discovery of what causes the disease.

If one does not know the cause, then one cannot provide specific treatment. Fortunately, we can do a great deal today without knowing why the disease develops.

Some of the same factors that are believed to cause the adult disease may be responsible for juvenile rheumatoid arthritis. But no one knows. It is all in the realm of speculation. As soon as we know why children get this chronic and potentially crippling disease, treatment will no doubt become even more effective.

THE BRIGHT OUTLOOK

In general terms, here is what you, as a parent of a child with rheumatoid arthritis, may expect during the years that lie ahead:

• More than half of the children will outgrow the disease. There is nothing inevitable about their fate. I see patients—a few now adults—who no longer have any form of the disease and are not receiving any treatment. But this is no guarantee that this state of affairs will continue. Another decade or two and then I can report to you what the 20- and 30-year outlook is likely to be.

At this time the outlook seems to be improving. In 1965, when I had treated these 100 patients for a minimum of five years, 48 had no disease. Now that I have finished 10 years of treatment, 60 patients are in remission.

• There is as yet no way for me to accurately predict what the future holds for each individual child. Those with an acute onset most often tend to develop disease in several joints; those with disease in several joints are likely to have this form of the disease for a good number of years; those with early symptoms of pain in only one joint tend to develop the least amount of arthritis, but a few develop pain in more than four joints.

• Even the mildest form of the disease requires careful, long-term supervision. Sometimes, years after the arthritis has disappeared, a subtle, symptomless eye disease (iridocyclitis) appears. Undetected and untreated, this eye inflammation may cost a child the vision in one or even both eyes. You must be watchful and make sure your child is regularly examined. For although the arthritis may be gone, the disease continues.

• Juvenile rheumatoid arthritis seems to run in families. I have encountered several instances of two or three children with this disorder in the same family. In one of my families, the mother and all three daughters have rheumatoid arthritis. Such familial "clustering" of rheumatoid arthritis is fairly well known. What is puzzling is that the degree of involvement differs so much among these four patients.

• Finally, the earlier you seek treatment for your child, the better the outcome. This observation is supported by a statistical analysis of my first 100 patients. There seems to be a significantly better outlook for the children whom I saw within one year of their first symptoms, no matter what type of disease they had. If you let three or four years pass by without vigorous and continuous care, then you may not achieve the best possible results. Proper care, given early enough—even when the disease is severe —pays off in long-term results.

It is high time that parents become more knowledgeable about the early signs and symptoms of the disease. Far too often, children who have had vague complaints, or even those mysterious and evanescent fevers, go untreated for months and even years. And this is a great pity! Their parents should have been more alert about the possible consequences. Such oversight or unintentional neglect can cause great harm. I have found that, invariably, parents are the ones who first spot juvenile rheumatoid arthritis. But they must take the initiative in seeing that their suspicions are confirmed by a correct diagnosis. Then, parents are the ones who are most concerned and responsible for the care and treatment of their child.

PARENTS ARE PARTNERS

I learned an important lesson from the parents of Donna Rafferty, the very first young rheumatoid arthritis patient I ever saw. I could not help her. But I could do a little something for her parents. I talked with them and listened to what they had to say.

The Raffertys lived fairly close to the medical center. Besides Donna, they had four other children. Like many young couples with a large family, they were in constant financial difficulties. Donna had been born at just about the time that Mrs. Rafferty had decided that there was only one way she could make ends meet. She had to have a full-time job; her mother would take care of the children.

This did not work out as well as expected. There was suddenly a great deal more friction in the family between the adults and the older children. Mrs. Rafferty came home from her secretarial job to find all manner of new problems she had not counted on. There was more money, but life, instead of becoming simpler, seemed more complicated. And then, when Donna became ill, the extra money did not help either, since Donna's medical treatments ate up every extra penny, and then some.

An even greater burden was more difficult to explain. Mrs. Rafferty, and to a certain extent her husband, felt somehow that Donna was their "neglected" child, just because Mrs. Rafferty had gone to work. This did not seem to be true. But that made little difference. Because of this neglect, the Rafferties felt a guilt they could not express. It took a lot of talking with them to get them to understand that juvenile rheumatoid arthritis is not due to what a parent does or does not do for a child. As we chatted daily, I was at least able to convince them that Donna's disease was not some sort of retribution. Instead of mourning a presumed misdeed, they needed to adopt a positive, helpful attitude. For once Donna could go home, they would be in charge of her treatment. Therefore, they had to be enthusiastic about giving drugs, applying heat, and doing exercises with the little girl.

Slowly their attitude changed. By the time they took Donna home from the hospital they had learned two important lessons: An ill child needs a good deal more support than one that is well; parents must constantly demonstrate that the illness makes no difference in their love. But they must not overprotect or spoil the ill child. What they need to do is to give a little more time to the child, to work with her, to show their love, not in words but in deeds—to make the periods of exercise or heat treatment a warm and loving moment, to avoid unpleasant, strained, or regimented feelings. I am always urging the fathers as well as the mothers to become optimistic partners in treatment. And should a father come home too late during the week to work with his child, he should take over for his wife when he is home during the weekend.

Perhaps the single most important lesson for parents to learn and understand is that the old saw about "Desperate diseases require desperate remedies" just does not apply to children with juvenile rheumatoid arthritis. In fact, the milder the treatment, the better the outcome. It has been my sad experience to see what happens when parents do not believe in this simple principle of treatment.

In Chapter I, I briefly mentioned the tragic fate of Rachel Warner whose parents were anxious for something dramatic and decisive to be done for their child, but were unwilling to work little by little to achieve the best possible results. Rachel's juvenile rheumatoid arthritis was first noticed when she was two years old. Hers had been a polyarticular onset, and she seemed to be doing quite well on aspirin, daily physical therapy, and heat treatments. The physical therapy was being done at the clinic's rehabilitation section, primarily because Mrs. Warner was unwilling or unable to work with her daughter at her home. So, complaining and resenting us, Mrs. Warner appeared daily at the clinic, except for weekends. This went on for about two years. The child was doing very well, although she had rather severe disease. The staff at the clinic also thought that they were beginning to win over the parents, so that more would be done by the Warners at home. One of the reasons we had insisted that Rachel be brought to the clinic as often as she was had been the extreme amount of doctor-shopping her mother had done before she had finally consulted me.

We had increasingly let the Warners do the exercises we had prescribed, although Mrs. Warner had trained her daughter never to tell exactly what was being done at home. We realized we had problem parents on our hands, but we felt certain time was on our side. That naive assumption was short-lived. For just about then, a national magazine gave fantastic publicity to a worthless Canadian drug that was being prescribed by a physician in Montreal.

No sooner had Mrs. Warner read about Liefcort than she snatched up Rachel and headed for Montreal. I should have known, for the last time I saw Mrs. Warner, she had mentioned the magazine article and I had been very firm in telling her what was wrong with the drug, a mixture of cortisone and hormones.

I had one more opportunity to try and reason with the Warners. Several months after they disappeared, they brought Rachel to me to show me how great she felt, how much better she walked, and what a good appetite she had—all of which convinced Mrs. Warner that I was wrong and that at last she had found the right thing to do for her child.

I was appalled by what I saw. As mentioned in Chapter I, Rachel was only seven, but she was already menstruating, she had developed breasts, and she suffered from a fungus infection of her toenails! I pleaded with the Warners to stop the Liefcort, but they refused to listen.

The family disappeared for about two years; they went to Florida and then Texas, certain that the combination of Liefcort and a balmy, even climate would benefit their daughter more than anything that could be done for her at an arthritis clinic in New Jersey. Surprisingly, they reappeared in the clinic one day, and not a moment too soon. For in addition to the other side effects, Rachel's hip bones now had necrosis (which means death) and portions were collapsing. First the child had to be weaned from the drug she had been taking for so long. This, in itself, took six months. Then we put Rachel back on her former regimen of taking aspirin and receiving physical therapy. Finally, Rachel had to have an operation to remove the destroyed bone and tissues of her hips. It took another six months before Rachel was no longer in pain and could walk again. It was a dreadful ordeal to put a child through, just so that some obtuse parents should learn that desperate diseases do not necessarily require desperate remedies.

Here, briefly, are a few principles to guide you during the treatment of a child with juvenile rheumatoid arthritis:

• Learn everything there is to know about your child's illness. Only then will you be thoroughly convinced about how much can be done, and how much you will achieve in helping your child. Knowledge will put an end to your fears about crippling, and will orient you to positive comprehensive care in which you are an active participant.

• Acknowledge early that aspirin is the best single medicine available for your child. If it works, accept no substitutes. But remember that your child will take large amounts of aspirin four or five times a day, and should your doctor require it, you may have to waken the child for another dose of aspirin during the night. Ignore people who downgrade this drug as being not "serious enough" for a disease as serious as rheumatoid arthritis. These people just do not know what they are talking about.

• Once the arthritis is suppressed, there is an inevitable temptation on the part of a parent to stop giving a child all that aspirin. But experience has shown that this is wrong. You must continue administering the prescribed drug, no matter what it is, for weeks or months before gradually withdrawing it. Under your doctor's orders, you will eventually give smaller and smaller doses. Do not do this by yourself.

• Balance rest and exercise: Don't overdo the rest, start the exercises while a child's joints are still tender and even painful. Don't overdo the exercising! Let your child rest, for proper rest allows joint inflammation to subside. But activity must follow, and soon. Don't wait for the joints to become completely free of pain before your child moves around. Keep in mind the old axiom, what you don't use, you lose! So as you encourage your child to be as active as he or she can be, also begin to make exercises a pleasant twice-a-day ritual. I cannot sufficiently stress the importance of exercise. It is the only way for you to maintain motion in your child's joints. By maintaining motion, you are doing the most important job of all, you are preventing the possibility of a joint becoming deformed. Deformity is, of course, the beginning of disability and crippling. Your efforts can help prevent deformity, and all you have to do is to work with your child in doing the simple exercises a doctor will prescribe for you. Just like prescribing aspirin, the regime of rest, activity, exercise, and heat treatment may seem awfully simple. But it is vital to the health and continued well-being of a child with rheumatoid arthritis. And the parents who work easily and well with their child are, in truth, full-fledged equal partners with a doctor. When parents are unable to work with their child, then the outlook is grim. In such rare instances, I insist that a child be brought daily to the hospital so that professional physical therapists work with the young patient. However, in the overwhelming number of families, the parents are perfectly capable of doing a top-notch job, and they can easily avoid the trouble and expense of daily trips back to a clinic and hospital.

• Pay no attention to suggestions about special diets. A

sensible, well-balanced diet is what your child needs. Only if a child with rheumatoid arthritis is undernourished will I suggest any vitamins or dietary supplements. By and large I have not found this necessary.

• Finally, continue to be informed about your child's illness, what you must do, and also what you can reasonably expect from treatment, and remember all this is a *gradual* learning and training process. Then, after you have become accustomed to your new duties and are relaxed about what the future holds for your child, it is time for you to become aware of a few nonmedical considerations that may be important.

A child with juvenile rheumatoid arthritis may be in need of a special school or specific tutoring. Some school systems are equipped with facilities and personnel to provide at-home instruction for the handicapped. Some of the new equipment is quite sophisticated and features closed-circuit television so that the child can see what is going on in the classroom as well as respond to questions. Some towns have phone hookups between the class and a sickroom. In some instances, the school will arrange for special transporation or for physical therapy as part of the school day.

If your child is hospitalized, check with the social service department of the hospital to see what they are able to do in providing special tutoring. You will lighten the burden of your child if he or she does not miss any schooling. In the hospitals where I have worked, the social worker made arrangements for tutoring. Occasionally, when a child went home, but was not physically able to go back to school, the tutor would then visit the home until the child could return to a regular school.

Once a child is well enough to go back to school, make sure to smooth the way. On occasions, I have done this, sometimes a social worker. But parents are just as effective. Smoothing the way means going to the school's principal or nurse and educating them about your child's disease. You will be surprised how often teachers are completely unaware that juvenile rheumatoid arthritis exists, and that the needs of these children are really very simple.

All you have to do—or get your doctor to do—is to explain the nature of the disease. I have always received and have never known anyone else to get anything but a very sympathetic hearing when the facts about a child's needs have been explained: A child is likely to have morning stiffness. Perhaps there is a certain measure of physical limitation, so that not everything the gym class does can be done by a child, but don't put too many, too unrealistic, or too stringent limitations on your child's activities. Consult your doctor about what your child can or cannot do. You might have to explain about the medication your child is taking and the importance of taking them at specific times during the school day. Invariably, it is the wisest course to be as open as possible with the school authorities.

In my experience, school personnel have been extraordinarily cooperative. I cannot recall a single instance when a child was excluded from school because of juvenile rheumatoid arthritis. But it is best to prepare the school so that there is no likelihood of misunderstanding or else the child is needlessly hurt. Occasionally, a teacher during the first few days of class has taken a child with juvenile rheumatoid arthritis in front of the class and explained what was the matter, and what a child had to do in order to remain as active as his or her class-mates. This worked, because suddenly there is no mystery. Everyone knows what is different about a particular child. It does not, apparently, cause any emotional trauma. It seems that full disclosure works with children. For the moment the entire class knows, there is nothing to wonder and whisper about. Once out in the open, the child is accepted, and what makes the child different is promptly forgotten.

At the New Jersey Medical Center, Mrs. Delta Boxer was the coordinator who specialized in smoothing the way for arthritis patients, young and old. She recently reminded me of several examples of what was happening to some of our first patients, when nothing was done to explain to the schools about their possible problems.

One child became very tired and listless, usually in the afternoon. One of her teachers interpreted this fatigue as "plain inattention"; the teacher would then scold the child who went home crying, and would not say anything to anyone. But her unhappiness about going to school was soon noticed. After the mother went to talk to this teacher and discussed the droopiness that assails some juvenile rheumatoid arthritis children late in the afternoon, the teacher scolded no more. In fact, a little rest period was permitted, and this half-hour made all the difference in the child's life. She stopped hating school, and once again loved her school and even the teacher who had scolded her.

I cannot emphasize how important it is to find such a small thing in your child's life and straighten it out. Unhappiness can actually be the trigger of an arthritis attack. The emotional stability of a child is vulnerable, just like the adult's, except the child will be much less likely to come and tell you very clearly what is causing his or her unhappiness.

Another little girl became extremely reluctant to go to school. Her mother thought it might be "school phobia," since she had read about that condition. But it was all very simple, and not a complex psychological problem. The child had developed arthritis of the hands, but her mother had failed to let the penmanship teacher know about it. Before the child became ill, she had been one of the outstanding students in that class. When she suddenly began to write very poorly or would not write at all, her teacher thought it was all due to "a lack of effort." She accused her former star pupil of being sloppy. This upset the child, who was unable to tell her teacher that she was easily tired and her hands felt stiff and painful. A five-minute discussion with the teacher took care of that problem to everyone's satisfaction.

A bright young man was having difficulty in his second year of high school. He had been an outstanding pupil, but after an attack of juvenile rheumatoid arthritis, it became difficult for him to concentrate. He applied himself as diligently as he had before he became ill, but somehow he was unable to absorb or retain what he was studying.

It was close to examination time when Mrs. Boxer finally learned about his problem. He had become extremely tense and anxious, afraid that he might fail his French exam and would not be promoted. But Mrs. Boxer saved the day. She called the principal of the high school who understood at once and had a conference with the other teachers. Without disrupting the school or the young man's life, a solution was quickly found. Special tutoring in French was arranged. And when exam time came, the young man was given more time to finish his paper work; in fact, if he felt tired, he was allowed to rest between exams.

This was enough to relieve the emotional tension. With the pressure off, and rest periods when he needed them, the boy passed all his examinations. He was promoted. All it took to bring about this happy ending was a little understanding and one 15-minute phone call.

Parents are frequently concerned about their own feelings about their child's illness. Many of them are angry that they are afflicted with the ills of their child. And when I notice this, I try to be as reassuring as possible. While I cannot stop parents from feeling as they do, I do try to reason with them about the effects their feelings might have on a small child who cannot understand a parent's conflicting emotions. Whatever you feel, don't give the child the idea that you are angry with him. The one thing you do not want to do is to handicap a child emotionally. The fact that the child has a serious physical disease is quite enough.

How do you prevent emotional crippling, when physical crippling threatens? It is not an easy thing, but it can be done. Being easy on yourself as parents and easy on your child will do. By working with a child and making it as enjoyable as if you were playing ball will do much to preserve a pleasant give and take. After all, you are not a doctor in a white coat doing something mysterious in a laboratory. You are a loving parent helping the child who needs you. This can be the most potent therapy, if you do it simply, easily, without fear or strain. I have seen fathers grow close to a young son whom they never really knew before as they were doing the daily heat treatment. Relationships have flourished, and as they have, so has the child. I have visited a home while a mother and daughter worked together, and I saw how this was a happy occasion with much playful teasing and many jests. And I was very impressed, since this helped the mother as much as the child.

Several of the parents have worried about disciplining their ill children. I generally suggest that they don't. Never strike a child—in fact, avoid any outburst or excess emotions. This is not good for the child or for the parent. If you are upset, don't take it out on the especially vulnerable, helpless child. One child I treated regularly used to have a bad flare-up of her disease after her mother and father quarreled bitterly. The father would strike the mother and occasionally the child as well, and within a few days after such wild family scenes, the child would be at the clinic. Sometimes, I would insist that the child stay at the hospital until the family situation calmed down.

One of the reasons I suggest that parents do not discipline children with rheumatoid arthritis is that the children confuse the disciplinary measures with a lack of love and support, something these children need extra large helpings of, especially when they are in pain or discomfort, or face the loss of their usual outdoor sports, or schooling, or other activities that were routine before they became ill.

And I also keep asking, "How naughty, how badly behaved can a child be that has an attack of juvenile rheumatoid arthritis?" The answer usually is not very! This is a time for tolerance, for letting discipline slide. The worst punishment might be having television watching time reduced. And, while I am on that subject, I urge parents to monitor what their children see, so that they do not become overexcited or upset. While I do not really believe that emotional upsets are as serious a trigger of attacks of juvenile rheumatoid arthritis as they are of the adult disease, I still believe in "cooling" it. Don't overstimulate the child.

At the same time do not allow the sick child to become the tyrant in the house. Be sweet, loving, yet firm. A child understands this, I believe, and will not feel deprived or unloved. Since the age range of children with rheumatoid arthritis is rather wide, there are no hard and fast rules that I can set down. As a parent myself, I find it unnecessary and unpleasant to be constantly scolding or saying no. But I do like to set reasonable limits on what can and cannot be done. And my child knows what is acceptable to me, and so does yours, I am sure. Teenagers are the ones that will find their disease most disheartening. It is very difficult to convince a 14-year-old cheerleader, ballet dancer, and all-around athlete that for the time being she had better stop these activities. But sometimes she can be interested in becoming a swimmer, and in investing the time and energy she formerly expended on three activities on only one.

Much to my pleasure and surprise, parents have managed to interest their children and themselves in activities that were new to them. Some children became more avid readers than they had been before. Other parents and their children started to go out more than before, to theaters, to movies, to museums, to performances of the opera, the ballet, or a symphony orchestra. It was fascinating to observe the horizons being broadened, and then, when the child was completely well again, the broadened interests remained. Reassuring also is the fact that the illness of a child often helps to bring families together—just as it can, unhappily, drive a family apart. But most often the close relationship established during the difficult periods of the illness were forged into permanent, beautiful ties that have lasted and have helped the children to grow and mature, while the parents take a particular deep satisfaction in being parents as well as successful partners in treatment.

IV. *The Silently Suffering Majority:*
My Patients with Osteoarthritis

Do you remember Mrs. Rosario, the first of those memorable patients who really taught me about being effective as an arthritis specialist?

As you will recall, I was puzzled and unhappy because Emily Rosario was not making any progress, despite all her show of sweet cooperation. It was the clever sleuthing of Mrs. Boxer, the social worker at the medical center clinic, that discovered why. It seemed that Mrs. Rosario had been convinced by her sister-in-law that nothing could be done. And so nothing was done, and for quite a while. Furthermore, both ladies had, for the sake of their arthritis, become gin-and-garlic devotees; this home brew they considered all the medicine they wanted.

In a sense, Mrs. Rosario's sister-in-law had a point in her cynicism about osteoarthritis treatment. On this even the experts agree. Drs. Bernard M. Norcross and Salvatore R. LaTona of the State University of New York at Buffalo School of Medicine have called osteoarthritis "the most mismanaged of the rheumatic diseases, usually as a result of undertreatment."

But rarely was there such undertreatment as in the case of Mrs. Rosario, who came to the arthritis clinic for companionship and turned to the bottle for the relief of her symptoms.

Unfortunately, this was no laughing matter. Mrs. Rosario had so-called "erosive" osteoarthritis. This is not a typical "osteo" form, since it causes fierce inflammation of the joints, especially the fingertips, which become warm, swollen, and very painful.

There is little comfort in telling patients with this kind of hand pain that "osteo" is far more common, but much less damaging, than rheumatoid arthritis, or repeat what all the textbooks state: There is little or no inflammation in osteo; this is a supposedly degenerative form of "wear and tear" arthritis. After all, these patients are in pain, and they are scared, because they are certain that they are inevitably going to be crippled. This is not true. But doctors just do not see this type of erosive osteoarthritis too often, and they are likely to agree with a patient who is afraid of having rheumatoid arthritis.

There are two dramatic differences between osteo and rheumatoid arthritis of the hand. Erosive osteo is a self-limiting disease; it stops. And the simplest way to tell whether you have osteo or rheumatoid arthritis of your hands is to observe whether your fingertips are involved. If so, this certainly suggests osteo. If your knuckles and finger joints nearest the palm swell and are painful, then this is probably rheumatoid arthritis. But be extremely cautious that this difference does not confuse you. Often enough I have seen doctors confused by these two very different diseases.

The name osteoarthritis is inappropriate and that is

why I usually shorten it to just osteo, which means bone. I do this because arthritis means inflammation of the joint, and most often there is little or no inflammation of joints in osteo. Other doctors prefer other names for osteo, such as degenerative joint disease, or arthrosis (a joint having limited motion), or even hypertrophic (overdeveloped from overuse) arthritis. But you need not trouble yourself with all these terms. You only learn from all these names that there are various forms of osteoarthritis, and little agreement on what to call them. The popular idea is that you get gray hair and osteo at about the same time. Supposedly, by constant use of your limbs, you eventually begin to wear out either the joints or what lubricates them.

Beware of such gross simplifications. Recent research suggests that osteoarthritis is more complex than the simple notion that cartilage and bone are just worn away or degenerate as you grow older. A recent survey found that osteo begins at about 25 years of age, not in middle age. Other investigators have suggested that the degeneration seen in osteo is not really wear and tear, but a matter of biochemical changes in the lubrication of the joint. As a consequence, the wear and tear concept seems to be losing ground to the more modern theory, the biochemical one.

But professional opinion is slow to change. Many experts still think that osteo results from a combination of growing old, from irritation of the joints, and from normal wear and tear. Chronic irritation of the joints due to overweight, poor posture, or continued strain from physical exertion is believed to be one of the main causes of osteo. But what makes me doubt the old theory is that enough research has now been done to indicate that the mechanical wear and tear theory may not be correct.

A group of New York investigators have shown that weight does not seem to be an important factor in the development of osteo. Also, they found no relationship between a patient's age and when osteo develops; they were impressed by the frequent presence of osteo in only one hip. If osteo is due to wear and tear, why would one hip become affected and not the other? This finding casts doubt on the wear and tear theory, but does not *prove* a biochemical cause. But I suspect future research might.

There is as yet no clear-cut answer to why people develop osteo; evidence suggests that there is probably no simple, single cause.

The biochemical theory of the cause of osteo implicates heredity, changes in metabolism, and also the endocrine functions of the body. Growth hormone or other hormones may be out of balance. But these concepts—until they are shown to be meaningful—are as helpful as the wear and tear theories. The biochemical theory of the cause of osteo happens to be more modern and more hopeful. For if the cause is something awry with the biology or chemistry of the body, then the development of biologicals or chemicals—medications or drugs—that will combat the disease process is possible.

Needless to say, the question of what caused her erosive osteo did not much trouble Emily Rosario. She knew generally that osteo is the most frequent of all arthritis complaints, with perhaps better than 50 million victims in this country. She also knew that osteo seems to be diagnosed almost always in older people—I am careful not to say "always" because I am not certain of this. Osteo is seen more often in women than men. Mrs. Rosario was well aware that the menopause is often the time of her life when a woman first feels the symptoms of osteo—pain and stiffness most often while using her fingers, hips, or knees. She traced her own troubles to the change of life.

It was not until we had managed to bring her sister-in-law to the clinic that Mrs. Rosario stopped being afraid that she would end up as a cripple. She began doing the very simple things I had outlined for her. She took aspirin and did the hot paraffin applications that I had prescribed as part of her daily treatment. (Some patients prefer electrically heated gloves.)

It was almost two years before Mrs. Rosario was feeling better. And then the pleasantest of gifts was granted her. Her erosive osteo suddenly stopped. She had suffered no deformity, and she has no further discomfort. When she comes to the clinic on occasion, she is just checked to make sure that she has no flare-up of her erosive osteo. Emily Rosario was extremely fortunate and knew it. An act of God, she called it. Actually, as I kept telling her to tell her friends, it was *that,* as well as the natural course of her disease.

Because osteo is a relatively mild disease, it usually can be managed with aspirin, physical therapy, and, if necessary, weight reduction, and when needed, orthopedic measures such as traction or a neck collar. If aspirin fails, more potent drugs (such as indomethacin or phenylbutazone) or the use of cortisone-like drugs in the affected joint are tried, but very carefully, since such drugs may cause unpleasant side effects. As you already know, all these drugs act to relieve pain and disability, but are ineffectual in stopping the disease process.

A drug that may be effective in counteracting the degenerative changes in osteo is high on the list of research priorities. The cartilage of patients with this disorder is thought to be deficient in chondroitin sulfate, a component of the ground substance of tissues. In theory, a drug capable of stimulating production of this substance would counteract the destructive changes that take place. But, as yet, none has been found. I look forward to the time when such a drug is finally available, because then we will have learned more about the aging process and how to prevent it. This is what makes research in osteo so very exciting. Among early findings are:

• In learning how joints develop in the fetus, it was found that movement in the embryonic stage of life plays an important role in their normal development.

• In the laboratory, a number of chick embryos were paralyzed, while others were allowed to develop normally to serve as controls. In striking contrast to the normal specimens, the paralyzed embryonic joint cavities failed to develop, became filled with fibrous tissue, and the joint surfaces were distorted. This research is the equivalent of producing osteo before birth, and again shows that osteo is not necessarily a part of aging.

• In mice, rats, or rabbits, new formation of collagen was shown to be a possibly basic cause of joint stiffness. Collagen is the chief constituent of the connective tissue found between the body's cells. Surgical removal of newly formed collagen from areas around the joints produced immediate relief of stiffness, but the long-term results were not satisfactory, because new collagen formed during the healing process.

• In man, there has been some research on how normal people walk, stand, and sit, and how their spine is affected as they move. No such study has ever been done before. From knowing what happens during motion and at different ages, this research seeks to provide baselines of what is normal, and so determine precisely what happens to the body as one ages or as one develops osteo.

This is important work, since little precise information now exists about what happens to the joints as they age normally.

These are a few examples of basic laboratory research. The importance and significance of these findings may not now be readily apparent to you or even to the investigators, but may be discovered as research proceeds. It is only one necessary aspect of the probings into the mystery of osteo. There are other advances being made on the clinical front. For instance:

• A substance has been identified that is capable of stimulating significant bone growth in adult dogs. This growth hormone is being studied for possible use in the treatment of osteoporosis, a condition associated with aging, in which bone "dissolves," becomes brittle and soft, and fractures easily. This is very valuable research, since 350,000 fractures a year in this country alone could be prevented if senile osteoporosis and postmenopausal osteoporosis could be eliminated. Osteoporosis is the reason some people over 50 develop backaches or why some older men and women appear to shrink in size. The condition is most prevalent in persons over the age of 60. However, recent surveys disclose that after the age of 35, 35 percent of the women examined and 19 percent of the men already have some degree of osteoporosis.

• Artificial replacement of the hip has been one of the most spectacular advances in the treatment of osteo in recent years. What was once a relatively long and trying operation has become quicker and safer. Thousands of people who previously would have been condemned by hip disease to a painful limp for the rest of their lives are now able to walk around without pain. But there is still a great deal of improvement in artificial joints to be made, particularly in making replacements of destroyed knees, elbows, and shoulders. Each of these is a "bio-engineering" project that requires the study of joint movement, of the strains the artificial joints will have to stand up to, and of what happens to metals or plastics used in surgery as they are worn down by continual friction or stress.

How about joint transplants? Not just yet. The answer is, of course, a matter of priority. People will die for lack of a new heart or a new kidney, but no one dies for lack of a new hip. There have already been pioneer joint transplantation operations, but not enough to know if this approach is sufficiently effective to be justified.

Osteoarthritis was first observed in man 500,000 years ago, but despite being such an antique malady, it is relatively new to research and a fertile field for discovery. There is a long list of questions that need answers!

Why does the normally smooth cartilage of one or more joints become progressively softer and less elastic, pitted, and frayed? Why do whole segments of cartilage disintegrate, exposing the underlying bone? This is what hurts and makes the joint hard to move.

Formation of bony spurs is one of the typical osteo signs, but no one really knows why they occur. This is another osteo mystery that must be solved. These bony protrusions, outgrowths, or spurs (called osteophytes) form at the outer edges of the joint and extend into nearby tendons and ligaments. Again, this is not only painful, but impairs movement. When a spur develops high on the spine, close to the neck, traction is used, often with considerable success. People wear a surgical collar as treatment for a bony spur that has developed as part of their osteoarthritis.

In severe cases of osteo, the disease may destroy the normal structure of a joint. Such cases, however, are relatively rare. Moreover, the ends of the bones do not usually grow together or fuse in osteo as they do in advanced cases of rheumatoid arthritis. That is why osteo does not cause severe, permanent crippling. However, when osteo attacks the hip, then, in some cases and especially among older people, trouble results. A good deal of function has been restored even to the elderly because of the successful efforts of research surgeons. Various types of surgery, arthrodesis, osteotomy, arthroplasty, or joint debridement —all of them discussed in the chapter of rheumatoid arthritis—are also used to benefit the osteo patient.

Osteoarthritis can occur in any joint, sometimes even the jaw bone. But why are certain joints more prone to become involved than others? The most commonly involved joints are those that bear weight, such as the hips, knees, and spine. Also frequently involved are the terminal joints of the fingers and joints at the base of the thumb and big toe.

But osteo seldom affects the knuckles, the wrists, elbows, shoulders, or ankles (joints frequently involved in rheumatoid arthritis) except when these joints are previously diseased or injured, or are subjected to repeated strain or injury that may occur while working or in the pursuit of athletics. There is yet no explanation of this. Why does strain affect one joint and not another?

The scientists who believe that osteo is related, at least in part, to the relentless wear and tear of joints, particularly the abnormally rough use of certain joints, often point to the fact that, in many cases, the specific joints affected depend on a person's occupation. Baseball pitchers and tennis players may develop osteo of the elbow, football players of the knees. Ballet dancers may get osteo of the ankles. Pneumatic-drill operators may develop osteo of the wrists.

Doctors tend to separate osteoarthritis into a "primary" and a "secondary" form. Primary osteo starts without any apparent triggering cause; secondary osteo results from injury or trauma.

Primary osteoarthritis is more generalized, occurs mostly in women and affects small joints, especially in the fingers. It occurs somewhat earlier in life, occasionally even in the late 30s and early 40s, and seems to be more common in some families than in others. Heberden's nodes, those bony enlargements of the end joints of the fingers and similar enlargements of the middle joints of the fingers, Bouchard's nodes, are most often observed in primary osteo that tends to be a family characteristic. But nodes also follow injury to the finger in secondary osteo, in conditions such as "baseball finger" or "bowler's finger."

Typical Heberden's nodes are multiple, appearing first in one finger and spreading to the other fingers. These nodes may be painless, but in some cases they appear rather suddenly with redness, swelling, tenderness, and aching. Patients with Heberden's nodes may complain of numbness and tingling of the fingertips, and "clumsiness" of the hands.

Although the enlargement of the finger joints can be painful and unsightly, good function of the hands can be maintained and crippling is not likely to occur.

Secondary osteo mostly strikes the larger joints (but also small joints if they are exposed to excessive stress), and occurs late in life as a rule. It is seen in young people only if a particular joint is badly abused—the arthritis of Sandy Koufax is a typical example.

However, whether osteo is primary or secondary, a fascinating and unsolved riddle is why some people have no pain at all, while others suffer constant nagging pain that persists even while they are resting or begins whenever they move after periods of inactivity—as in getting up in the morning. The pain is caused by irritation and pressure on nerve endings, and bears little relation to the amount of joint damage. I have seen patients with severely affected joints who have less pain than those patients with mild osteo.

I am constantly aware of this curious phenomenon and also of the great variation in the way people feel pain. You may ignore pain, someone else may exaggerate it.

Among my osteo patients there is Mrs. Katherine Schreiber, a lovely, charming, and cultured lady who I suspect is over 80, but who looks much younger. She lives alone in a comfortable apartment. Because of her extensive osteo of the spine, she should have pain and be severely limited in her activities. Instead, she does her housework, goes out shopping, and attends concerts or the opera she so loves. Her mornings are sometimes difficult because her back and knees hurt and feel stiff. However, a small amount of specific exercises, her hot tub bath in the morning, and a capsule of her prescribed medication (indomethacin) help her feel limber eventually.

I am always disturbed by the large amount of swelling present in her knees and the degenerative changes of her neck and lower back. Also, she does not take her medication as regularly as she should, and is unable to shed the 40 pounds of excess weight that I thought was aggravating her arthritis.

But despite all of this, Mrs. Schreiber is holding her own as the years pass. She does so because she does not have the amount of pain I would expect her to have, or she simply does not feel the pain as strongly as someone else might. On the occasions I see or speak to her, I admire her determination and self-reliance, her capacity to be interested in the world around her. She appears younger than she is because of her young outlook. She really is quite wonderful.

She is unlike Julia Rykes who is somewhat younger than Mrs. Schreiber and who has a mild osteo problem. I have to see Julia every week in order to provide enough reassurance to keep her active. If I miss seeing her once, she will sit at home all week and brood, claiming that I have abandoned her. She will stop all treatment, eliminate the aspirin, the warm tub baths, neglect her housework, or any other chores that she is perfectly capable of performing. Yet, she has mild disease. Is it the attitude that makes the difference between Mrs. Schreiber and Julia Rykes? I think it is.

A positive "nothing can get me down" attitude makes the difference in whether you are old or young. How you live your life is likely to be how you experience your arthritis. For example, though osteo is supposed to be a disease of middle or old age, I have had patients who were quite young. Nina Bergman was only 32 years old when she first felt pain and stiffness of her lower back. She also had pain that shot down from the back of the thigh to the knee. This is a type of nerve inflammation called sciatica. A tall, slender, and attractive woman, Nina was troubled by worries about becoming crippled and the fear that she would be unable to care for her husband and two small daughters.

All her diagnostic studies proved to be normal, except for the X-ray of the lower back. It seems that she had been born with abnormally shaped sacral bones at the bottom of the spine; these bones apparently were putting undue stress on the lower spine. Small spurs and outgrowths (osteophytes) had developed. One of the spurs was pinching the sciatic nerve and this caused the pain in her thigh. Such pain is called "referred," that is, a problem in one part of the body is felt somewhere else where no problem exists.

Episodes of back pain would come and go every six months or so, and would trouble Nina for two or three weeks. But once she understood the mild nature of her arthritis, she relaxed and forgot her fears. Her management is very conservative: she takes aspirin regularly and uses a heating pad for 20 minutes during the day. Even when troubled, she manages her usual routines. You cannot tell any difference between Nina Bergman and any other attractive, suburban housewife. Even after four years of osteo, despite her recurrent back pain, she continues to lead a normal life; except, to get enough exercise she has organized a gym class each morning with some of her friends. Here is another typical example of arriving at a proper attitude. Remember, you are not born with the right attitude. But once you know about your osteo, you can easily develop a nice combination of concern for treatment and a determination to go on living that is the most successful way of dealing with osteo.

Prevention of osteo is a possibility. Do you have a vague back problem? Does your hip ache? Is one leg shorter than the other? A job that causes stress or trauma to your body? If this is so, something can be done *now* to keep the condition from getting worse. There are so many kinds of things that may be troubling you that there is not enough space here to go into every possibility. Typical of the kind of prevention that may be useful is the building up of one shoe if you have one leg that is shorter than the other. If you have some sort of joint pain, see your doctor in any case even if you think you are too young to do so; he can suggest ways and means whereby a simple problem will not develop into a serious form of osteo. You might have to exercise, perhaps even try for a different job, if the one you now have causes the kind of physical stress that will prove troublesome later. Whatever may be necessary may well be justified if it prevents problems later.

If you suspect you have osteo, by all means see your doctor now. By consulting him you will find out if a painful joint is really due to early osteo or something else. Remember that most often you will need very little treatment to make you feel better.

A careful analysis of your symptoms and a thorough examination of the aching joints should give a doctor a fairly good idea of what the problem is. Laboratory tests are not as necessary to confirm the diagnosis as to rule out more serious problems. A useful test, the ESR (erythrocyte sedimentation rate), that measures how fast blood cells settle to the bottom of a small tube. Normal sedimentation rates are seen when you have osteo, but no complicating illness. Sometimes blood counts are done at a first examination, and at frequent intervals when your doctor prescribes drugs that may cause side effects. Occasionally, a detailed analysis of joint fluid may be done. The most valuable "diagnostic test" in osteo is an X-ray, and no thorough examination is complete without it.

One of the complicating illnesses a doctor usually checks for in his first examination of a patient with osteo is diabetes. This is particularly important if you are under 40. Recent studies have shown that young diabetic patients have osteo more frequently. But what this means is not clear at this time.

Unfortunately, much is as yet unknown about osteo-arthritis. Still, enough is known so that the most popular current misconceptions should no longer live in the present. Osteo is *not* inevitable. There are people over 90 who do not have any symptoms. Neither is osteo a problem exclusively limited to the Geritol set.

It is a safe bet that with all the various kinds of research into the cause and treatment of osteoarthritis that not too many years will pass when something can be done about its process. In the meantime, there is effective treatment that alleviates most of the suffering caused by man's oldest physical enemy. Osteoarthritis laid low the mighty dinosaur 200 million years ago and began bothering Pleistocene man a mere 50,000 years back. Although progress has been slow up to now, there is some comfort in that it has accelerated to practically breakneck speed. It's been a long, long time, but, at last, we are beginning to learn something about this, perhaps our most ancient, enemy.

V. *The Oldest Complaint: Rheumatism*

> The rheumatism is a common name for many aches and
> pains, which have yet got no peculiar appellation,
> though owing to very different causes.
>
> WILLIAM HEBERDEN, 18th-century physician

THE FIBROSITIS PATIENT I love best is the lady who has me
at her beck and house-call, my darling wife, Josephine.

I am pleased and proud when my wife says that I am
her favorite doctor, not because I am her husband, but
because I have done so much to take the annoyance out
of the rheumatism that causes her repeated aches and
pains. You see, the girl that I married is fibrositis-prone,
and so are a lot of other people. They suffer from rheumatism.

All that I have read suggests that rheumatism is probably man's oldest and most common complaint. And like
the oldest profession, rheumatism lacks status. This is
perhaps so because the forms of rheumatism that I am
about to describe are, with one exception, more annoying
than serious. They tend to be ill-defined, imprecise,
poorly understood conditions that often are likely to go
away without any treatment. Since the "conquest" of
rheumatism appears to offer no vast financial gain or research glory, no one is really investigating these condi-

tions to learn more about what causes them and too few doctors are trying to learn how to improve treatment.

Most people who have rheumatism hesitate to ask their doctor about it. Doctors in turn tend not to listen, either because they can't hold still for anything as insignificant as a little rheumatism, or because they feel unable to do anything about the problem.

I firmly oppose the do-nothing approach, and because I do I am not only appreciated in my home, my popularity has spread to our rather large family. At any one time, I am likely to be treating several relatives for muscle ache or some sort of pain that is definitely not arthritis but rheumatism. And what I do for the rheumatism of those who are closest to me is really very simple, so simple that you can probably do most of it quite effectively for yourself.

PAIN-CAUSING QUARTET

Of the four major forms of rheumatism, bursitis is probably the best known, even if the bursa are something of a mystery to most people. They are small connective-tissue lubricating sacs that are found between muscles, tendons, or any bony prominence in hundreds of different places throughout the body. It is not too far-fetched to liken the bursa to the sand bags that once protected or cushioned buildings and other structures during air raids. Bursa seem to serve a not too dissimilar shock-absorbing function for the body.

In addition to bursitis, there are three other familiar conditions, which are strictly speaking "rheumatism." Each is an inflammation of a specific non-bony part of the human anatomy. Rheumatism need not be confused with arthritis, if you remember that arthritis is an inflammation essentially of the joints. Rheumatism refers to the inflammation of various kinds of soft tissues that insert into the joint, lie adjacent to it, or support or surround a joint.

Don't be confused by the term soft tissue. Some of these are fairly tough and hard, such as the tendons, which are fibrous bands that connect the muscle to bones; an inflammation of these white strips is called tendinitis. Muscle inflammation is called myositis (myo meaning muscle); a dangerous form of myositis that seems to attack only older people is polymyalgia (much muscle pain) rheumatica (due to rheumatism).

Terminology in rheumatism tends to be vague or to overlap: fibrositis is an inflammation of any type of fibrous tissue, most often the outer layer or sheath of muscle. To abet confusion, muscular rheumatism is also called fibrositis. There is hardly any difference between myositis and fibrositis, other than the suggestion that myositis is a more complex or deep-seated muscular disorder. As you have no doubt noticed by now, wending your way through the labels used for rheumatic disorders is very much like working your way through a maze. Because all forms of rheumatism are poorly described or understood, the various forms tend to blend one into the other. They are as unavoidable as death, and far more antique than taxes. They are the grab-bag of conditions (primarily fibrositis, myositis, or tendinitis) familiarly known as the "miseries" or "rheumatiz."

There is lumbago which is a form of fibrositis of the lower back. And you probably know many types of tendinitis, vague "agues and plaints" due to injury or strain, which are popularly called typist's finger, chauffeur's shoulder, tennis elbow, mailman's or soldier's foot, housemaid's, nun's, or rug cutter's knee, and even weaver's bottom. It may interest you to know that the last named is caused by long sitting on hard surfaces, and is more formally known as ischiatic tendinitis or ischiatic bursitis. It is almost impossible for a doctor to tell the difference between these two conditions. There is inflammation of either the tendons or the bursae at or near the bony prominences of the pelvis—the parts that stick out the most where you sit—the ischial tuberosities.

My profession is fairly notorious for neglecting its own—shoemakers' children going unshod—but I feel strongly about paying attention to my wife's recurrent bouts of fibrositis. Hers is a minor malady, to be sure, but also extremely annoying and exasperating.

FIBROSITIS AND MYOSITIS

Fibrositis makes you feel achy, sore, and stiff, and so does myositis. In fact, much that I have to say for one condition applies to the other.

Most often, you have a sudden attack of fibrositis at the wrist; sometimes you feel pain at the base of the neck— this is the well known "wry neck" of torticollis. Fibrositis also occurs at the shoulder or near the knee. Fibrositis may also be generalized, so that you feel a vague but distinct discomfort throughout the body. This tends to be a chronic and recurrent condition. Some people—my wife is one—seem to be predisposed to both localized, acute attacks and repeated, chronic fibrositis.

Primary fibrositis, the type that exists by itself and occurs spontaneously and for unknown reasons, may be subdivided into the acute and chronic forms. Most often, an acute attack does not become the chronic condition. The acute type of fibrositis starts suddenly and departs swiftly. Attacks may come on in hours and disappear in days or within a week or so. As the name implies, the chronic condition creeps upon you slowly over a period of days and even weeks, and then may last for weeks or months. Chronic conditions seem to recur more frequently than do acute attacks. Occasionally, a neglected acute attack does become chronic.

Whether acute or chronic, when fibrositis is localized, it affects a comparatively small area—known as a "trigger point." The base of the neck is a particularly common trigger area. Dr. Janet Travell, who was the official physician to President Kennedy, became famous for her understanding and treatment of fibrositis trigger areas. She taught her patients to spray these areas with a topical anesthetic called ethyl chloride. She also injected the trigger points with procaine, a pain reliever.

There is a secondary type of fibrositis that accompanies, precedes, or is caused by some several hundred diseases. Perhaps the most familiar form of secondary fibrositis is the unpleasant and vaguely painful muscular condition that you get with or just after an attack of the flu or other viral infections. You rest, take a little aspirin, and it disappears. Fibrositis symptoms also accompany many types of arthritis, and particularly plague rheumatoid arthritis patients. Sometimes, the presence of fibrositis complicates a definitive diagnosis of rheumatoid or other forms of arthritis. As you will learn in a subsequent chapter, secondary fibrositis may be the only, as well as the earliest, telltale symptom of an occult cancer, one that is as yet to be detected and diagnosed.

Patients with fibrositis are often quite unhappy because they have gone from doctor to doctor without receiving much help. They have not even received any assurance that they have a mild form of rheumatism.

The fear of crippling looms large in their minds. Fre-

quently, doctors who cannot help them actually do injury
to these patients by suggesting that their vague aches and
plaints are imaginary, emotional, or "psychological."

Fibrositis should not be confused with psychogenic
rheumatism, since it is very easy to differentiate between
fibrositis and psychogenic rheumatism. People with psychogenic rheumatism don't just complain of aching, stiffness, or soreness. As Dr. Hugh Smythe of Toronto has
pointed out, these people describe the symptoms of their
psychogenic rheumatism in rather dramatic and bizarre
terms—they use emotionally loaded metaphors. For example, a patient will say, "My pain burns through my left
breast and out through my back." Pain has acquired a
symbolic meaning; such patients are not as much victims
of rheumatism as they are victims of a number of mild to
severe psychologic disturbances.

Treatment of Acute Fibrositis

The most important thing you can do for yourself is to
do something about the pain. Take two or three aspirins
at least four and possibly up to six times daily.

If aspirin provides no relief, then it is time to see your
doctor. He may prescribe a combination of propoxyphene
and aspirin (Darvon compound 65) to be taken four
times daily, or Empirin Compound No. 3 with codeine,
one or two tablets every four hours as you need it. If
aspirin upsets your stomach, then Darvon alone or
acetaminophen (Tylenol) with or without codeine may
work. These drugs relieve pain.

If they, in turn, do not help, then your physician will
try indomethacin (Indocin), a drug that you have read
about before because of its effectiveness in reducing inflammation. Another alternative is phenylbutazone (Butazolidin).

Many of my patients prefer that I inject "trigger points" of their fibrositis (or bursitis or tendinitis). Sometimes the injection alone will do the trick, and no further medication is required. I tend to give both the short-acting pain reliever lidocaine (Xylocaine), and a steroid drug (Decadron with Xylocaine). Your doctor may prefer one or the other, or some other injectable adrenocorticosteroid preparation. But you must be warned of one very curious phenomenon. Occassionally, you will experience a "post-injection flare-up." This means that your pain will get a good deal worse than it was, but then as swiftly as it appears, it vanishes. I warn all my patients about the risk of this "it may get worse before it gets better" phenomenon. Very few refuse to have a trigger point injected, and only a small proportion experience the flare-up.

Don't hesitate to rest in or out of bed for a day or two if it makes you feel better. Although fibrositis and myositis are not serious conditions, they may prove quite exhausting. I think this is a matter of how you experience pain. Some people are worn out from a little pain, while others tolerate a surprising amount. It is a very subjective thing, and you must decide for yourself whether your fibrositis requires you to take it easy. Often, if you call what you have by its formal name, that is, fibrositis, people will more readily understand if you take to your bed briefly. They might not be so sympathetic if you just say you have a vague muscular pain.

Immobilization of the affected limb or part of the body may make you feel more comfortable. For instance, having your arm in a sling may help rest your painful shoulder.

All the various heat treatments will help to make you feel more comfortable. Apply moist heat packs for 20 to 30 minutes twice a day. It also might help to take warm showers or tub baths, or to use an infrared heat lamp for half an hour. But make sure that the lamp is 30 inches away from your body. Massages may also help, but they must not be done too vigorously. Some doctors also recommend the moderate applications of ultrasound, but I am not at all convinced that this does any good.

Much to my surprise, my friend Dr. Nathan E. Headley, an arthritis specialist in Los Angeles, finds that local applications of cold, moist packs, or stroking with ice, may actually prove to be more effective or beneficial than heat treatments, especially if you use the "cold treatment" within the first 24 to 48 hours after feeling your first fibrositis symptoms. One way to do a cold treatment is to wrap an ice bag in a thin towel and place it on the affected area as you would a hot-water bag. Leave the ice bag there for 20 to 30 minutes; do this twice a day. Another technique recommended by Dr. Headley is to gently stroke the involved area with an ice cube for 5 to 10 minutes or until the acute pain or spasm subsides. This you can do every 15 minutes, or every hour, until you feel no more pain.

Treatment of Chronic Fibrositis

For people who have chronic and recurrent fibrositis, the best medicine is often the sincere assurance that they do not have a potentially serious deforming or crippling disease, or that they are not on their way to getting something worse—osteoarthritis, for instance. This information has an astonishingly salubrious effect.

My wife, who had been consulting doctors for years and was not really disturbed—perturbed would be a better word—worries no longer and now accepts the fact that she is going to have perhaps three acute fibrositis attacks a year, and every other year some chronic fibrositis. I think it has been extremely helpful to her that her family does not make a great deal of fuss when she has fibrositis. Her understanding (and ours as well) has done much to help her cope better with the annoyance she feels when her fibrositis strikes. It also seems to me that her attacks are shorter when I insist she go to bed whenever she feels most uncomfortable. She is not coddling herself, but treating her rheumatism. By going to bed, she really rests. Whenever she feels she has too much to do to allow her to take to her bed, she soon finds out that the fibrositis lingers on. Then she realizes it is a lot more beneficial and sensible to treat her fibrositis at once than to attempt to ignore it.

In the chronic condition, the previously mentioned pain relievers will be helpful, as is Indocin. Other anti-rheumatic or anti-inflammatory agents, such as the ones used in rheumatoid arthritis, don't seem to be required in chronic fibrositis. There is little need for drugs like cortisone or narcotics other than codeine (and codeine only when necessary). This is, after all, a very benign or mild disorder.

Do apply any of several forms of heat as you would during an acute attack; cold treatments do not seem to help in the chronic condition. But exercises will. Do them right after you have applied some form of heat. It seems to me that what exercises you do is not as important as that you are moving about so that your muscles do not lose their tone or begin to atrophy: inaction will make muscles lose their full size or waste away a little. If your symptoms get worse two hours after you have done some exercises, that means they were too strenuous. Don't stop, but do fewer, less strenuous ones, for slightly shorter periods of time. Finally, make sure that you avoid excess fatigue or exposure to inclement weather. In other words, coddle yourself a trifle until you are over your fibrositis.

When Feet Defeat . . .

Foot fibrositis is quite common, quite uncomfortable, and quite unnecessary. But far too few people who complain bitterly of aching feet are aware that the smartest treatment is simple prevention. All you have to do is avoid unnecessary strain and stress. You can't keep off your feet. But you can avoid the three major stresses that cause most of the foot fibrositis. Lose weight if you are too heavy, try not to become depressed or stay troubled too long, and don't get carried away by your sense of chic. Each may compromise the health of your feet.

There is no need to explain why being overweight puts pressure on your feet; there is after all only so much your feet can support. But you may not be aware that your aching feet may be telling you that you are emotionally upset. It all has to do with the way people walk, according to Dr. René Calliet, a professor of physical medicine and rehabilitation at the University of Southern California's School of Medicine. He says we stand or walk the way we feel, and I believe he is right in thinking that when a person is depressed, a flat-footed gait with no spring in the step results. This is a kind of stress feet were not meant to absorb. Fibrositis may be the penalty.

High fashion produces some very strange footgear, but that is not as hard on the feet as the tendency of some ladies to opt for the smallest possible size of shoe, one that provides the least amount of support. You will do your feet a favor if you balance your footgear between what is in fashion and what makes sense. Go barefoot, wear sandals as much as you can and the climate allows.

Foot fibrositis is every bit as painful as it sounds, and it is best avoided. If pain persists, by all means see your podiatrist or foot doctor. Either he or your regular doctor might provide you with an injection of the trigger point of your fibrositis. But before you ask for this, try aspirin or other pain-soothing products. Remember that steroid injection of a trigger point sometimes causes a post-injection flare-up, and that is especially unpleasant below the ankles. Long-term preventive measures are best. Better yet, remember, your weight, your emotions, your footgear may all conspire to defeat your feet.

BURSITIS AND TENDINITIS

These two conditions, one the inflammation of bursa, the other of tendon, can be discussed together because they look and feel the same, and are treated similarly. Sometimes they even occur together. Other than for purposes of a precise diagnosis, it usually does not matter which you have.

Both are miserable, causing pain, swelling, hot and "exquisitely tender" discomfort. Just try to move the elbow or shoulder, or whichever part of the body is affected. Howls of pain may accompany the slightest motion. Nonetheless, both forms of rheumatism will subside by themselves, usually within a week or two, even without treatment.

No one can pinpoint the exact cause of an attack of acute bursitis or tendinitis. I find that if I ask a patient enough questions, he or I can pinpoint something that triggered the attack—an injury or extra strain due to some sort of overuse. But some people are especially susceptible to attacks of bursitis or tendinitis, and they should do things in moderation, whether at work or at play. People who play golf are prone to tendinitis of the wrist, those who play tennis get it in the elbow. Attacks occur usually after they have played too long or too hard. Handball players not only get tendinitis of the elbows, but also in the wrists and shoulders.

Diagnosis is usually easy. You can usually put your finger right on the spot where the tendinitis or bursitis hurts.

X-ray is important in diagnosis, particularly when the tendinitis or bursitis is calcified. However, most attacks are not associated with calcium entrapment in the area of tendon or bursal inflammation; flecks of calcium, therefore, will not be apparent on the X-ray of the involved part. Your doctor may take X-rays of both elbows, for example, when only one hurts. He does this in order to compare one elbow with the other; this is especially important when calcification is present.

Most attacks of tendinitis or bursitis will subside spontaneously, even without treatment, usually within a week or two. But some will not. If you consult a doctor right away, you may save yourself a great deal of discomfort; I would certainly not let more than ten days go by without seeking treatment.

I think that one of the best reasons for getting medical help with these conditions is the unpredictable nature of an acute attack. It may linger on and may become chronic so that you will develop an immovable or "frozen" shoulder or a "frozen" elbow, for which you will have to have specific treatment, injections, and increasing amounts of exercises to help you regain the lost motion of these joints.

POLYMYALGIA RHEUMATICA

In New Jersey in 1961, I first saw Martha Jacobs, a pleasant, jovial white-haired lady of 68 who had been troubled for over a month with aching and stiffness of the shoulders, upper arms, and hips, particularly in the morning when she got out of bed.

Prior to the beginning of these symptoms, Mrs. Jacobs had been in excellent health, busy with her frequent visits to her 41 great-grandchildren, all of whom lived in Jersey City. Now, suddenly seized with aches and pains, she thought she was doomed to become crippled. Her problem had puzzled two physicians before she was admitted to the hospital.

When I first examined Mrs. Jacobs she had the full range of motion of her joints. There was no swelling. The muscles around the shoulders and hips were tender to touch, but her muscle strength was excellent.

The usual routine laboratory studies were normal, except that the value of one of the tests, the erythrocyte sedimentation rate, was extremely high. The high ESR was helpful in dismissing the possibility of fibrositis, since the test is normal in this disease. X-rays were normal. And so was a biopsy of the skin and muscle taken from one of the tender areas of the arm.

After a thorough review, one of my interns, Dr. Gerald Levey, suggested that here might be a disease that had received considerable attention in the English and European medical journals but was unknown here.

Dr. Levey was right; Mrs. Jacobs had polymyalgia rheumatica. But we could only be certain after we had done a number of laboratory tests to rule out two other serious considerations—cancer and a muscle disease called either polymyositis (much muscle inflammation) or dermatomyositis (when a rash accompanies muscle inflammation). The major difficulty here is loss of strength of muscles, particularly around the shoulders and hips. Inflammation of the muscles causes an outpouring of muscle enzymes that can then be detected in the blood and measured—muscle enzyme tests confirm polymyositis. But, because there was no inflammation of muscles in Mrs. Jacobs's case of polymyalgia rheumatica, these tests proved normal.

Cancer also had to be ruled out, and it was necessary to perform a number of studies to make certain Mrs. Jacobs was not harboring a malignancy somewhere. All this was tedious, but it was the only way to be certain.

Mrs. Jacobs turned out to have typical, although then rare, polymyalgia rheumatica. Most patients are women over 60. Their aches are generalized, but occur primarily in the muscles and soft tissues at the shoulders and hips. Why this happens in the elderly is unknown. Some patients have more extensive symptoms; they may complain of great fatigue, fever, anemia, and loss of weight.

Polymyalgia rheumatica lasts for only a few months, but occasionally aches and stiffness linger for a year or two. The condition is self-limiting, as it was in the case of Martha Jacobs. Her condition cleared up within a year, and she has had no recurrence since then.

Mrs. Jacobs's condition was so unusual that Dr. Levey and I described it in an article that was published in *Arthritis and Rheumatism*, the official journal of the American Rheumatism Association. Since our report of 1963, there have been over a hundred medical journal articles on this disease in this country. But the disease is not as simple as Dr. Levey and I, or the European physicians who had written about it earlier, first believed it to be. From studies of large numbers of patients, it is now

apparent that polymyalgia rheumatica can be complicated by inflammation of the small blood vessels of the
brain. Temporal arteritis (inflamed arteries of the side of
the forehead) occurs in one-fourth of all patients. If undetected and untreated, the arteritis can rapidly lead to
blindness. I have seen at least a dozen patients who have
gone blind from this disease, simply because physicians
did not know about the association between the achy
muscles and this treacherous blood vessel complication.
For the blindness can come rapidly, in only a few days.
And once this happens, blindness is permanent. To prevent this complication, cortisone-like drugs are used for
three to six months.

In a fashion typical for a rheumatic disease, nobody
can quite decide what to name it. Confusion reigns, since
polymyalgia rheumatica is also known as polymyalgia
arthritica, peri-extra-articular rheumatism, anarthritic
rheumatoid disease, peri-arthrosis humeroscapularis,
myalgic syndrome of the aged, senile arthritis, and peri-
articular rhizomelique. There is, as you may have noted
while reading this chapter, room for vast improvement in
our knowledge and treatment of various forms of rheumatism. One advance, however, would really be staggering. If rheumatologists could only agree on what to call a
disease!

VI. *Male Liberation: The Conquest of Gout and Ankylosing Spondylitis*

IF ONLY TODAY's feminists would turn their furious attention on the major forms of arthritis. What wonders they could achieve! What a marvelous women's march on these diseases it could be! What pressures they could exert on men to improve treatment techniques and to make them widely available! What research they could stimulate!

I indulge myself in this fantasy because arthritis in all its major manifestations is so horrendously unfair to women. They pay a fearful price. And no job discrimination, nor any old-fashioned double-standards of morals and behavior so victimizes the fair sex. Many more women than men suffer from rheumatoid arthritis, osteoarthritis, and various forms of rheumatism. Even the little girls are not spared, since they, far more often than boys, suffer from juvenile rheumatoid arthritis. And as adults, the ratio of those racked and hobbled by this disease is five to two in woman's disfavor. To my knowledge, there is no explanation for this appalling predilection. It is simply a totally unfair phenomenon.

Adding insult to injury is the rosy picture in the almost exclusively masculine forms of arthritis, gout and ankylosing spondylitis. And it was a woman who helped achieve a recent and notable advance in the care of gout. Co-discoverer of Zyloprim (allopurinol), a major drug used widely to prevent severe attacks of gout, was chemist Gertrude B. Elion.

The outlook for gout and for ankylosing spondylitis is indeed sanguine. Gout was recently called "one of the most satisfactory of the rheumatic diseases to treat." In ankylosing spondylitis, vast strides have also been made in recent years. The only solace I can offer women while reporting all the "good news" for victims of gout and ankylosing spondylitis is that the small number of women who get these diseases respond to treatment as well as men do. Rarely does either sex develop both diseases at the same time.

Of 100 gout patients, 95 are likely to be men over 30. The five women are usually older; women tend to get gout after their menopause. A similar ratio applies to ankylosing spondylitis. There are nine times as many men as women spondylitics, and they are usually between the ages of 15 and 35.

Both these forms of arthritis are disorders of younger people, although once in a while they strike a child or attack an elderly person.

FAREWELL TO THAT RED, HOT, SWOLLEN TOE

There they sit, fat and uncomfortable in a big arm chair, resting an enormously swaddled foot on a cushion. This depiction of gout victims is provided by cartoonists and satirists of 18th-century England, probably poor, starving wretches who envied those stuffed, prosperous men who suffered from gout. For centuries, gout has been considered the consequence of overindulgence and related to high and riotous living and drinking. But gout victims, often royal or intellectual, or both—men such as Martin Luther, Philip II, William the Conqueror, George IV, Isaac Newton, Benjamin Franklin, Theodore Roosevelt—were not invariably live-it-up types. Sometimes they were downright ascetic.

After centuries of being falsely accused of gluttony, boozing, and rich living, redress has come. Diet does not cause gout, and even if it did, today's drugs permit doctors the pleasant task of forbidding only a very few and unusual foods. Those low-protein diets doctors used to impose on highly resistant and resentful gout patients are no longer in use. Eating all that starch and sugar was, I suspect, probably as bad as the gout, for patients gained much weight, and the diet did little good in preventing gout attacks.

Today's gout patient may now indulge his supposedly classic penchant for indolence, carousing, and high-style dining to a remarkable extent. (The gout patient's life style may actually be a sign of his wisdom—high uric acid values have long been associated with greater than average intelligence.) What is held out in other forms of arthritis as a possible promise for tomorrow is available to gout victims today. Acute attacks, even in severe cases, can now be prevented.

At this moment, every doctor has an impressive arsenal of sophisticated, even elegant, drugs at his disposal. With them, he can control the painful inflammation of gouty arthritis as well as permanently reduce the level of the uric acid in the blood. For approximately one million patients who suffer from gout, this is tantamount to the conquest of their disease. We can now also prevent the formation of uric acid kidney stones, a complication that used to kill a great many gout victims.

For a better understanding of gout, let me explain the significance of these therapeutic achievements in terms of eliminating acute gout attacks as well as subsequently providing specific treatment for a number of problems as they may arise during the course of the disease.

Arthur Newton, a slim and handsome man of 35, a witty and talented writer, had felt a sudden sharp and darting pain at the base of the big toe. He suspected right away what it was. Gout was a "family" illness. Grandfather Newton and one of Arthur's uncles had suffered from excruciating pain because of their gout. Grandfather had died of kidney failure as a result of his gout. And he had been in terrible pain before his death. He had suffered from grossly distorted hands and feet that were riddled with huge chalky deposits of hardened uric acid. These are the characteristic tophi of gout. What actually killed Grandfather were deposits of uric acid accumulated in his kidney. These are similar to the chalky material in the tophi of hands and feet. But in the kidney the urate deposits prevent function, often with lethal consequences. Two generations ago, of course, little could be done for such a patient except ease the pain of the acute attack. And up to ten percent of patients died after years of having this major form of arthritis.

Arthur's uncle had a somewhat different and more pleasant experience. At first, his hands had become distorted and crippled because of the enormous deposits of uric acid. However, about twenty years ago, he started receiving a drug that not only reduced the tophi of his hands, but also prevented the formation of new ones. This was the first uricosuric drug (a uric acid reducing agent), Benemid (probenecid). As a matter of fact, the uncle had been one of the first to have improved on the new drug and his doctor had made him a present of some before-and-after photographs that were hanging in his study. The before picture showed hands that were obviously swollen, distorted, and unfit for use. The after photograph showed the hands virtually normal.

So my patient came to me knowing that he would not have his grandfather's experience. But Arthur wondered whether he would have to suffer the way his uncle did. Would he have recurrent attacks? His first terrible pain in the toe had made him ready to go on a very stringent diet.

I had some pleasant surprises in store for Arthur. There would be no strict gout diet. I suggested that he not eat certain foods—innards, like sweetbreads, liver, and brain, and fish delicacies like anchovies and caviar. These should be avoided since they are rich in purines. And the more purine you consume, the more uric acid you form. Uric acid production is, however, only part of what has gone wrong in gout.

Gouty arthritis is caused by two possible biochemical mechanisms of the body: There is a vast overproduction of urates, the main chemical substance in uric acid, or the kidney is unable to get rid of the uric acid via the urine. Some gout patients have only one of these metabolic defects, some have both. They are born with the defect and have inherited their predisposition toward developing gout. However, to be producing a great deal of uric acid is not a sign of gout. Some people have a good deal of uric acid in their blood but do not develop gout symptoms.

There may be several reasons for this. The older you get, the higher the uric acid; if you take one of a long list of drugs, your uric acid will rise.

Two to six milligrams per 100 milliliters of blood (expressed as mg. percent) is within the normal range of uric acid values. Some experts in the gout field tend to treat anyone for gout who has a blood uric acid above nine mg. percent, even if he does not have any arthritis at all. Treatment will presumably prevent the impending acute attack. Preventing acute attacks is even more important for those who have had one.

And, of course, that was the best news I had for Arthur Newton. His first attack could very likely be his last.

In his case, I really did not have to wait for the results of the blood test, or take X-rays, or remove material from his toe to see if there were crystals of urate present. The suspicion that he had gout was very strong, just on the basis of his painful toe and the facts of the family history. I did not delay treatment to wait for the results of the lab tests, since I had one other method of determining if this was really gout. I prescribed colchicine for Arthur. If he responded, then I knew for sure he had gout. Colchicine is rather specific. If it doesn't work, then it is usually not gout.

After explaining all this to Arthur, I began to map out for him what the future was likely to hold. In gout, you and your doctor must consider two methods of attack. You must first deal realistically with the acute episode. Then you make plans for long-term management.

TREATING ACUTE GOUT

I explained to Arthur that during the acute attack we would forget the underlying mechanism of his gout.

What we wanted right now was to relieve the acute inflammation in his big toe. At that particular moment, the control of high uric acid levels is unimportant, and could only lead to complications. For attempts to lower the levels of the uric acid in the blood are likely to prolong the acute attack. This happens because you are mobilizing the uric acid throughout the body, and doing this might cause crystals to induce inflammation in other places besides the big toe. It is too much of a risk to take. So first things first.

To relieve the acute inflammation, we have three highly effective drugs, colchicine, phenylbutazone, and indomethacin.

If I suspect gout and the evidence is as good as it was in Arthur's case, then I start with colchicine. Colchicine was known in ancient times, but it was that famed gout victim Benjamin Franklin who introduced the drug to the United States. Just recently, research by Dr. J. Edwin Seegmiller, a distinguished former investigator at the National Institute of Arthritis, now at the University of California in San Diego, and another famed researcher, Dr. Daniel J. McCarty of the University of Chicago Medical School, have shown how colchicine works.

The swelling, incredible pain, and exquisite tenderness of Arthur Newton's toe appears to be due to the action of white blood cells, the leukocytes, that try to do something about the urate crystals that have become deposited in the joint fluid because of too high a concentration of uric acid in the blood. In their attempt to engulf the crystals (this process is called phagocytosis), the white blood cells produce a by-product that prolongs the build-up of the crystals. The inflammation continues. Dr. Seegmiller has called this a "self-sustaining, self-augmenting chain reaction." This can last for days or go on for months. There are long quiet periods; but repeated attacks, if untreated, come on more frequently and become increasingly more painful.

The reason colchicine is so effective for an acute gout attack is that it diminishes the ability of white cells to migrate into the area, and also prevents them from releasing the substances that produce the inflammation after they engulf the urate crystals. The drug provides a chemical interference (more formally, a block of chemotactic factor release) which prevents the inflammatory processes from becoming self-sustaining. The attack subsides.

Colchicine is still regarded as the best drug to terminate the excruciating pain of an acute attack of gouty arthritis. One tablet of the drug is given every hour, either until the patient experiences some beginning relief of pain or colchicine side effects such as nausea or diarrhea occur. No more than 12 tablets should be given for any single gouty attack. Experience has taught me that if 12 tablets do not work, more won't help. After the initial loading dose of up to 12 tablets, two or three tablets daily are continued for four or five days or else an attack may suddenly recur. Since the drug is also frequently used to avoid future attacks, the doctor may advise a patient to take the two or three daily tablets indefinitely. In some cases, during an attack, the physician may inject colchicine directly into a vein.

If colchicine does not work, then the diagnosis of gout must be questioned. However, colchicine may be ineffective when a gouty attack has been present for more than four or five days. For some unexplained reason, a few days' delay may make the gout colchicine-resistant; the longer you wait to take colchicine for an acute attack of gout, the less likely it is to work.

Although nonspecific for gout, phenylbutazone (Butazolidin) and indomethacin (Indocin) are also effective in relieving the acute gouty arthritis attack. Once the diagnosis of gout is established, then your physician may have you use any one of the three effective drugs either separately or, once in a while, two together. Occasionally, corticosteroids are given either by mouth or injected directly into the involved joint.

At the time of his first attack, I taught Arthur to carry his medication with him so that he could treat any subsequent attack at his first twinge of pain, the so-called "joint-warning" signs, as Dr. Thomas Weiss, a gout expert from New Orleans, likes to call them. These are a peculiar sensation of numbness, tingling, burning, stiffness, or dull aching—like a toothache—seldom severe enough to prevent using that joint. These signs of an impending attack are usually the same with each subsequent attack for that person, although there are individual differences.

When you are being maintained on two or three colchicine tablets each day, and you feel an impending attack, then take colchicine hourly, as if you were having a full-blown acute attack.

LONG-TERM MANAGEMENT

Colchicine will treat and prevent acute attacks of gouty arthritis, but they will do nothing to correct the underlying defect, the excess stores of uric acid present in the body's tissues. For this, other drugs are needed. There are now two types that will rid the body of its extra urates: The uricosuric (uric-acid lowering) drugs, probenecid (Benemid) and sulfinpyrazone (Anturane), or allopurinol (Zyloprim), a drug that blocks uric acid formation rather than reduces it.

It is sometimes difficult to get a gout patient to understand the difference between taking care of the acute attack and the long-term task of preventing subsequent attacks by doing something about what causes the gout. As I explained to Arthur Newton, the metabolic defect in purine metabolism or in uric acid excretion, or both, does not occur in animals, who seem to possess an enzyme called uricase, which acts to break down the uric acid so that it is eliminated in the animal's urine. Because man lacks this enzyme, the minute amounts of uric acid that normally circulate do not easily dissolve in the body fluids. That is usually no problem—the body maintains a proper equilibrium in all biochemical matters; and ordinarily there is only a tiny amount of uric acid in the body. The amount has been estimated at one gram, of which half is excreted each day. Gout patients, however, end up having perhaps twenty to thirty times the normal amount of uric acid in their body. This is accompanied by hyperuricemia, the elevated blood uric acid. Not all hyperuricemia is brought on by the inborn, metabolic defect. The defect in purine metabolism is often accompanied by the inability to excrete the purine breakdown product, the uric acid. A good many healthy men are believed to have elevated uric acid levels. These may be predisposed relatives of gout patients who have taken drugs, alcohol, have fasted, or eaten certain foods that contain high levels of purine. But that is not gout unless you have arthritis or kidney stones.

And then there is pseudo-gout, first described 40 years ago, but largely forgotten until Dr. Daniel J. McCarty revived interest in this condition in which calcium, rather than urate crystals, is deposited in the joint. The disease is different from gout, because large joints like the knee are usually subject to an acute attack. Colchicine is ineffective. Indomethacin and phenylbutazone are preferred in treatment of the acute attack, while injections of steroid solution are used in the chronic form of pseudo-gout (more formally, chondrocalcinosis).

But there are conditions that cause secondary gout: These are blood diseases, such as polycythemia in which the patient manufactures too many red blood cells, or leukemia in which too many white blood cells are manufactured. Certain bone diseases cause secondary gout, some of which have been linked to alcoholism. Lead poisoning has been linked to secondary gout; this has occurred in children who have eaten lead-base paint or in adults who have drunk moonshine made in stills when either the vats or the pipes were lined with lead or had lead soldering that dissolved in the alcohol.

After Arthur's initial acute attack had subsided, we had to come to some sort of decision about his long-term management.

Should his uric acid levels be lowered? There are several facts to be considered before you put a man on life-long drug therapy for gout. Does he have deposits of urate crystals in his joints, the tophi of tophaceous gout? Does he have frequent acute attacks? Is there any evidence of renal (kidney) damage? Is his blood uric acid above nine mg. per 100 milliliters?

Several of these criteria were met in Arthur Newton's case. But far too many patients are taking drugs to lower their uric acids when they have no symptoms of arthritis.

What I prescribed for Arthur was probenecid (Bene-mid), one of the uricosuric drugs that lowers the uric acid by promoting excretion rather than reabsorption in the kidney. By keeping blood uric acid levels near normal, crystal deposits are prevented and acute attacks are avoided, as is damage to joints and kidneys.

Arthur Newton knows that he must take Benemid indefinitely, since there is only prevention, but not cure, for gout. Every few months, he comes for a check-up to see that his uric acid levels are down, that the drug is working effectively. During the past five years, our treatment aims have been achieved. Arthur takes his drugs, and comes in for a six-month check-up. He has had no further acute attack and his blood uric acid level is under control.

But should something happen to trigger another attack, or should his blood uric acid shoot way up, Arthur knows that there are some other drugs we can use. Sulfinpyrazone (Anturane) is another uricosuric drug like Benemid. Should he develop very large tophi, he knows that they can be removed surgically. But there is little likelihood of his need for any change in treatment. During the time that Arthur has had gout, a new, rather different drug has been developed.

This is allopurinol (Zyloprim), which acts to decrease the production of uric acid, rather than increase its excretion. As I have mentioned before, promoting the excretion of uric acid may help to distribute the urate compound in the body so that deposits are formed. Allopurinol has been widely hailed as a great advance, because by blocking uric acid production, uric acid stones are much less likely to form in the kidneys or urinary tract. Gout patients who have kidney problems have greatly benefited from the discovery of allopurinol by Burroughs-Wellcome chemists George H. Hitchings and Gertrude Elion.

Arthur does not need allopurinol. But the day may come when he might benefit from this potent new drug. It is very reassuring to know that there are other medications to turn to in case his condition gets worse.

Because the drug is still relatively new, not all of its side effects have been fully studied. It may cause a fairly troublesome rash in patients with severe kidney problems, who are also the ones who need this drug the most. At this time, therefore, I reserve allopurinol for those patients who absolutely need it: Those with extensive tophi, those who can't take other drugs or for whom they have stopped working, and patients whose gout has led to severe kidney trouble or uric acid stones.

The future looks bright. As a recent pamphlet, prepared by the National Institute of Arthritis and Metabolic Diseases, points out, "It is possible that extensive research currently being conducted in clinical centers and laboratories throughout the world may result in identification of other basic defects which underlie gout. Such a finding could lead to more effective methods of treatment, and, hopefully, to an ultimate cure for this ancient disease."

PREVENTING THE POKER BACK OF ANKYLOSING SPONDYLITIS

The other young man's disease that can be effectively treated is ankylosing spondylitis. This disease is, as the name implies, a progressive condition in which the vertebrae (spondyles) are inflamed (spondylitis) and then become fixed in position (ankylosed). Untreated patients become "poker-backed."

A great deal can be done for the patients with this disease. But in contrast to gout, for which drugs achieve remarkable results, the patient must be prepared to achieve his own prevention. He must be convinced that he is on a permanent do-it-yourself project. He must be active and exercise, exercise, exercise.

In the case of Frank Farrell, whose emotional problems were discussed in Chapter I, the greatest obstacle to treatment was his refusal to spend three half-hour periods a day on his exercising. These exercises were simple. He did not have to use a gym, but could do them at home, in his office, or even in a hotel room if he was on one of his frequent trips. His failure to do his exercises was not because they were either complicated or inconvenient. He refused to do his exercises because he could not face the fact that he had a chronic, potentially crippling disease that might interfere with or wreck his career.

However, once we were able to get through to him, Frank did everything to help himself—he became a cooperative and eventually successful patient. No one looking at Frank Farrell today, many years after his disease started, would suspect that here is a man who without his exercises would probably be hunched over, unable to look anyone straight in the eye without lifting his head like a turtle.

Yet, how often have you seen a man with a curiously hunched-over stance? Often they are older, in their 50s or early 60s; sometimes they are surprisingly young. Pitiful is the word that best describes a man with neglected or untreated ankylosing spondylitis.

The disease is believed to attack five men out of every thousand, so that there are probably a half-million or more men in this country who risk developing the curious back deformity that is the stigma of neglected or poorly treated ankylosing spondylitis. One of my friends whom I have treated for the disease told me that whenever he waits at a street corner, he not only looks at the girls as they pass by, he also counts spondylitics. He claims his highest count was twenty men with early to late disease once while a girl kept him waiting at a corner in New York City for 45 minutes one sunny spring afternoon. He also could not bear to see the hunched-over conductor on his commuter train appear so uncomfortable day after day, as he bent over to collect the tickets. Finally, he spoke to the man. The conductor had never heard of the disease, and had accepted his discomfort and stoop as inevitable. He was grateful to my friend who had told him about ankylosing spondylitis.

That is step one—to be aware that the disease exists. Too few people and even too few doctors are. And this is important, because a correct diagnosis early and treatment as soon as possible achieve wonders in preventing the typical bent-over look.

This is a disease that primarily affects the back. Backache is frequently the first symptom. However, it is not the inevitable first sign of the disease. The first twinges of pain, or some swelling, may be felt in the hips, knees, or heels. Interestingly enough, although no pain is felt in the back, some "silent" changes may be beginning.

Richard Elliott was only 13 years old when he had swelling of his knees and pain in the right hip and right heel. His doctors thought he had juvenile rheumatoid arthritis because of his age. But when they took X-rays of his hips, his sacroiliac joints (which join the sacral part of the spine to the iliac portion of the pelvis) revealed changes that suggested the real diagnosis.

Erosion or wearing away of the bone and what looks like a spreading apart of the sacroiliac joint are the two sure signs of ankylosing spondylitis. That is why X-rays must be taken to make the diagnosis.

Actually, Richard did not feel any discomfort in the areas where significant changes were taking place. In fact, it was three years before he felt the classic back pain. By that time the aspirin he had been taking had helped reduce the swelling of the knees, and the pain in the hip and heel. When his back pain began, I switched

Richard to indomethacin (Indocin) since the aspirin no longer provided enough relief. That was seven years ago. Richard continues to take this medication. He is periodically checked for any possible side effects of this drug. But between indomethacin and the exercises for spine extension and chest expansion, he manages to lead a perfectly normal life. He also has not a trace of stoop, and is a nice looking 23-year-old.

Richard Elliott's silent and symptomless sacroiliac changes are typical of ankylosing spondylitis. Just as characteristic is a distinct loss of chest expansion. This also can be seen in patients much before they have any pain, and is a telltale clue.

The simplest way to detect the loss of expansion is to take an old-fashioned tape measure and measure the circumference of the body at the nipple line. Then take the same measurement after a deep breath is held. Normally, the difference between the normal and expanded chest is 2½ inches or more. However, in a young man with ankylosing spondylitis, the chest expansion is likely to measure less than one inch.

Here are some other early, telltale clues of ankylosing spondylitis:

• If the back appears curiously flattened out, it may have lost its normal curvature from spasm of the big muscles of the back.

• If a young man holds his knees straight while trying to touch the floor with his fingertips and he can reach only to his knees, he is likely to have limited spine flexion due to the disease.

• If a physician presses with his thumbs hard against the areas in the lower back where the sacroiliac joints are, the pressure he exerts will cause local pain, or pain in the buttocks. If an X-ray is then taken, it will reveal changes in the sacroiliac joints.

• If inflammation and spasm of the upper spine is present, the ankylosing spondylitis victim will be unable to stand with his back flush to the wall and then touch the back of his head to the wall without feeling a good deal of discomfort, if not pain; some are unable to do this at all. However, after drugs and exercises, they can; therefore, this is often a very easy way of measuring the progress made.

These early signs are not all seen in the same patient at one time. At best, a patient will have one or two such early symptoms that should not be neglected. For early treatment invariably provides a great deal of improvement, and the very *simple* treatment consists of balanced rest and activity, postural training, and therapeutic exercises.

FIRST, EASE THE PAIN

No currently available drug will cure ankylosing spondylitis, or prevent such complications of the disease as recurrent attacks of red, painful eyes (acute iridocyclitis), a widening of the aortic valves of the heart (aortic insufficiency), and amyloidosis, a potentially lethal condition in which the cells are infiltrated with "starch-like" particles.

But there are a number of drugs that sufficiently relieve pain and spasm so that the patient can start exercising. The drugs found effective are the following: aspirin in mild, early disease, phenylbutazone (Butazolidin) and oxyphenbutazone (Tandearil) for moderate to severe spinal discomfort, for which indomethacin (Indocin) is also useful. However, indomethacin is the drug that I have used most often. I believe that if clear-cut relief of even severe symptoms is not achieved by either phenyl-butazone or indomethacin, then the patient may not have ankylosing spondylitis. Again, as in other major rheumatic conditions, oral steroid drugs should not be taken, except when chronic iridocyclitis or inflammatory narrowing of the blood vessels (vasculitis) complicate the disease.

Muscle relaxants, gold injections, antimalarial drugs, or any narcotic or pain-relieving drug are not as effective as the drugs mentioned and should be avoided. That goes also for radiotherapy, irradiation of the spine. This old method of treating ankylosing spondylitis has not just fallen into disrepute, it is dangerous! It may cause leukemia even fifteen years after treatment is given. Ironically, better relief of pain can be obtained with drugs than with radiotherapy.

THE HEART OF TREATMENT

I never stop being amazed at what exercises can do for the patient with even advanced ankylosing spondylitis. Edwin Caplan, a very successful 48-year-old businessman, came to see me, cane in hand, tottering somewhat, and really afraid to cross the street since he couldn't see too well in front of him. He was a rather short, plump man, and since he leaned forward very badly, he seemed even shorter than he was. His apprehensive looking up at people was the worst part of his condition, as far as he was concerned. He had constant pain, but that did not bother him as much as his curiously vulnerable position in relation to other people. He did not need to tell me that, for the tragic consequences of being old before his time, bent and frightened, were all too obvious.

Incredibly, within two months of taking phenylbutazone, using heat treatments, adhering to new postural techniques, and performing his specially prescribed therapeutic exercises, Edwin Caplan was erect again. This was no miracle. It was what you can expect from simple, conservative treatment. To Ed, however, it meant having his full life restored.

He walks without a cane, is back at work running his business and, most important of all, he and his wife are having normal sexual intercourse again. When he first came to see me, he alluded to the fact that he was no longer a man but a hopeless, helpless cripple, a burden to his wife.

It did not take much talking to him to discover that he had stopped all sexual relations with his wife, as his back pain became increasingly worse and the flexion deformity of his spine increasingly made him feel "crippled." I urged him, right from the start, while he still felt discomfort in his back and hips, to try intercourse while lying on his side. At first he was reluctant to try this, but then found that this position was satisfactory to him and acceptable to his wife, as was the supine position, in which he would lie flat on his back. As he improved, and his back straightened up, Ed felt free to try previously preferred positions. And he knows that whenever his back bothers him he need not curtail his marital relations.

Because ankylosing spondylitis primarily affects young men, I always try to reassure them about continuing sexual intercourse. I have dozens of patients for whom the disease at first disrupted their sex life; but then, just a little modification in their sexual technique helped restore the pleasure and also avoid unnecessary discomfort.

THE WONDER OF THERAPEUTIC EXERCISES

There is a great satisfaction in looking at Edwin Caplan's before photograph and the one taken of him two months after treatment. Even better is to see him today, breezing into my office—ten years after he timidly hobbled in, disturbed and fearful, tentative and unsure of himself, and not quite trusting the support of his cane. The magic transformation between then and now is contained in the five words: Postural training and therapeutic exercises. Anyone can do it, and at any age.

POSTURAL TRAINING

The ankylosing spondylitis patient has to really rethink the way he sits, stands, and walks. He must constantly counteract the inclination, brought on by his disease, to bend forward and to stoop.

Occasionally, I will put braces on a man to promote good posture, but most often this is quite unnecessary. Almost immediately, patients follow my advice to consciously stand as erect as possible, and to walk and think "tall." This means he must avoid stooping, leaning forward, or bending over. Should Edwin Caplan drop a book to the floor, he keeps his back straight as he picks it up. He never lounges in a well-cushioned arm chair, but sits up in a chair with a hard, straight back. At night, he sleeps on a firm mattress that has a wooden bedboard underneath. He uses no pillows for his head, and he long ago gave up putting pillows under his knees (they used to hurt less when flexed that way). The drug he takes faithfully keeps him comfortable. At the beginning he tried all the usual heat treatments. Nowadays he takes a warm shower daily to help lessen the early morning stiffness.

It is the carefully prescribed exercises that literally have straightened him out and keep him that way. Only at the very beginning was he put in traction to help realign his neck; this was not as complicated as it sounds. Ed needed traction only for a few weeks, and it was done at home for half an hour, two or three times a day.

THERAPEUTIC EXERCISES

These are not just the cornerstones of treatment, they have become an intrinsic part of Edwin Caplan's daily life. Within a week after he saw me, and although he still had some pain, spasm, and inflammation, he had already been to a physical therapist to learn what exercises he was to do for 30 minutes three times daily.

He stands in a corner, with one hand against each wall at shoulder level. He next bends his elbows slightly, pulls his stomach in, and slowly leans forward to force his chest toward the corner. He then returns to his original position and repeats the exercises from ten to twenty times.

It is unbelievable how important this simple exercise is to Ed's treatment. It combines two important therapeutic principles—spine extension and chest expansion. Lying down or standing up, Ed does exercises that stretch his spine backwards, that is, in the direction that opposes his stoop. He works on his breathing and chest expansion because when I first saw him, he could expand his chest less than one inch. This forced him to breathe through his stomach, his chest breathing was too shallow because of his restricted expansion. His stomach had lost tone and he had developed a potbelly because he stooped and was forced to do "stomach breathing." He began doing various breathing exercises, including blowing up a beach ball. These exercises restored normal chest breathing. By doing them, Ed began to achieve a number of things. He could breathe normally, and he could pull in his stomach, and this enabled him to stand straighter.

From the beginning, all Ed's exercises were tailored to his specific needs. The physical therapist taught Ed specific exercises that helped to improve the functions of his hips and shoulders.

Sports activities were included in his exercise program. I made him give up a few things he loved, such as bowling and golfing, and suggested instead that he try swimming, archery, and racquet-type games like badminton or tennis. Actually, he really liked only swimming, but that was fine, because swimming causes the chest cage and spine to move and also limbers up the shoulders and the hips. As a matter of fact, Ed most often practices his spine-extension and chest-cage stretching exercises in the pool, so that swimming has now taken the place of most of his therapeutic exercises. He uses the back stroke to maintain full spinal extension and to avoid chest cage restriction. Other patients, who do not have as much motion of the shoulder as Ed has, cannot do the back stroke, but do a side or breast stroke.

Not being allowed to play golf, now that he looks and feels better, is a matter of annoyance to Ed, but he understands that golfing promotes flexion, rather than extension, as do bowling and surf-casting. As a compromise, I've suggested that he use a long putter and that he restrict his golfing to a driving range, so that he avoids long, tiring walks. Ed does not fish. Patients who like fishing are allowed bait- and fly-casting, or trolling, but not surf-casting because it imposes too much of a physical strain.

Exercising must be part of properly balanced rest and activity. After all, an ankylosing spondylitis victim has a serious systemic disease. He requires eight or nine hours of sleep every night. When possible, he should also get a short rest period in the afternoon in order to prevent general fatigue, as well as the tendency to droop in the late afternoon.

Ed is fortunate because he can take a nap on the couch in his office. Other patients who work as laborers may have to change jobs, particularly if they must do a great deal of lifting of heavy objects. Very few of my patients have had to give up their work or change jobs. Most often, they have managed to assume other duties at work, tasks that do not cause excessive physical strain and fatigue.

Richard Elliott, who came to see me at the very beginning of his disease, and Edwin Caplan, who had neglected his ankylosing spondylitis for at least a decade, are both doing very well now. To maintain their present status, they have check-ups four times a year.

Like them, the majority of patients with ankylosing spondylitis today can regain and maintain satisfactory physical function. They can pursue their usual routines with a minimum of discomfort or interruption from their serious, systematic, chronic and potentially crippling disease.

But there are those patients who do not respond to conservative treatment. These are the truly neglected spondylitics who are badly bent, in as bad or even worse shape than Edwin Caplan was when I first saw him. Gerald Kent was such a patient, and when he was still badly bent over after six months, the possibility of surgery was discussed.

SURGERY—A SUCCESSFUL LAST RESORT

Gerald Kent was 35 years old when he came to see me. His disease had begun rather insidiously in 1941 when he first had recurring low-back morning stiffness, and pain would wake him during the night. But nothing much was done for him, even in 1954 when Gerald complained of feeling weak, of having lost his appetite, and having dropped 40 pounds. At the time, he also had pain of the right hip. Four years later when I saw him, he was a curious S-shape, a posture due to the fact that he was flexing his knees slightly as well as stooping over, all the while attempting to hold his head up. There was nothing very unusual about any of the laboratory tests and his X-rays revealed typical changes. None of his peripheral joints, such as knees or shoulders, were affected. But he did have extensive flattening of the back, and was extremely bent over. For six months, all the usual conservative treatment approaches were tried, but to no avail.

That is when reconstructive surgery was discussed with him. And because he had seen the success we had achieved in a few other patients who had undergone spine surgery, Gerald Kent agreed to this complex and tricky procedure. Before attempting surgery, however, Gerald understood that he was about to undergo an extensive and delicate operation that could cause serious complications if unsuccessful, and if successful, requires a full year of aftercare, including wearing a full-body plaster cast for six months and then a metal brace for an additional six months.

What was done for Gerald seems rather simple in the telling, but is complicated in the doing. The surgeon removed a segment of the bony parts of the spine. Then, while still on the operating table, the spine is hyperextended, or literally cracked back to an upright position. Fortunately, no blood vessels or nerves were injured. Gerald won his gamble. Today he stands straight and erect, although his back is rigid, so that he cannot bend over normally. And he has to squat erect to pick up an object from the floor. But this limitation of function does not concern him, since he no longer stoops. Of all the ankylosing spondylitis patients I have mentioned, he is the only one in remission, so that unlike Frank Farrell, Richard Elliott, or Edwin Caplan, he no longer requires any medication. However, he continues to exercise, and returns for his regular check-ups four times a year. He feels that his trust in surgery and the year of aftercare paid off handsomely. However, his surgery would have been unnecessary, he now realizes, if only he had received treatment shortly after his disease began. He could have achieved the same results from early conservative medical care.

VII. *Arthritis Rare and Perplexing*

NOTHING IN MEDICINE is forever. What is considered a rare, dreadful, and serious disease today is tomorrow taken for granted as dangerous no more.

This has been the hopeful process of most of medicine. And this has been true in rheumatology to a remarkable extent during the past few decades. "When I was a student 45 years ago," wrote the eminent British physician Lord Cohen of Birkenhead, "nobody cared, and practically nothing was known of the genesis of the rheumatic diseases, and where there is ignorance there are many flights of fancy."

For the doctors who specialize in arthritis and rheumatism, ignorance has given way to insight; flights of fancy are being replaced by facts and data. They have learned about a vast number of rheumatic diseases—and are forever seeing a new one that neither they, nor possibly anyone else, has ever seen before. As the field becomes more learned, and more people specialize in some of its many aspects, some system of preserving all the accumulated knowledge must be set up. One of the methods is the establishment of formal training standards as well as the passing of examinations before a doctor can call himself a rheumatologist. The formalization of the sub-specialty of rheumatology is about to happen.

But there are major problems in making what arthritis specialists now know available to other members of the medical profession. Only half of the approximately one hundred medical schools in this country have departments or teachers to instruct medical students about the latest advances in the rheumatic diseases. And there is no burning passion to improve this situation, as Dr. Evan Calkins of the State University of New York at Buffalo, discovered when he was president of the American Rheumatism Association. In 1969, he made a survey of what heads of departments of medicine of the nation's medical schools thought about the present status and current importance of rheumatology—that is, the medical specialty of arthritis care.

The answer came from 76 men who, like Dr. Calkins, are in charge of departments of medicine at university medical schools. His results suggest that rheumatologists must first educate fellow professionals.

For the answer given by half of those who replied, all of them in charge of teaching medicine to medical students, was that arthritis specialists are "highly desirable, but not necessary." Arthritis experts were rated far less important than specialists in other diseases. Only skin specialists and allergists were deemed less vital.

Besides improving its own standards, rheumatology thus faces several awesome tasks. It must change the attitudes of powerful professionals who influence medical teaching, and who are also responsible for improved patient care, as well as for the research that provides most of the medical advances in arthritis.

Yet rheumatology has already shown what it can do. For, in addition to the significantly improved treatments already described, much has been discovered and understood about the rare and dreadful forms of arthritis that once inevitably doomed their victims. For these patients, more and more is being done. That in itself shows the importance of the arthritis specialist.

As you already know, arthritis runs its course throughout the world. But as you may only be beginning to realize, rheumatology, as shown by the conditions I am about to discuss, does something more. It is seemingly involved in all of medicine.

SYSTEMIC LUPUS ERYTHEMATOSUS—SLE

SLE and other disorders like it are the special province of immunologists, who study how the body resists disease. These experts have shown that SLE is an autoimmune disease. SLE victims are allergic to themselves—specifically to their own connective tissues. As yet, no one knows why SLE develops.

Considered one of the most serious rheumatic disorders, SLE is a generalized systemic disease that may affect any of the body's connective tissues. It is a disease that primarily affects young women, of whom an estimated twenty percent are stricken in childhood.

Since SLE primarily affects connective tissue, it strikes at the framework of all the body's vital organs, the heart, kidneys, lungs, blood vessels, and the brain. The disease is at its most serious when the connective tissues of the kidney become involved. When this happens, drug therapy, unsuitable to other forms of arthritis, is used and often with considerable success.

The steroid drugs, the very ones to be avoided in rheumatoid arthritis unless there is a specific, pressing need, are used lavishly. Huge amounts are given to SLE patients during acute attacks that include disturbed emotions or nervous breakdowns that resemble bizarre psychotic attacks. Steroids, which in huge overdoses may by themselves cause a psychosis, have been found enormously useful in counteracting the emotional instability of SLE. The drugs may indeed be life-saving, according to lupus specialist Dr. Naomi Rothfield of the University of Connecticut School of Medicine.

Dr. Edmund L. Dubois of the University of Southern California School of Medicine is one of the country's foremost lupus experts; he has had some experience with other drugs that can be used for the SLE patient, such as the antimalarials, the cytotoxic, and immunosuppressive agents. There is as yet no specific therapeutic agent for SLE; treatment is variable and really depends on the severity of symptoms. Dr. Dubois has found that often *no* treatment is necessary in patients who have little wrong with them other than some arthritis, a false-positive syphilis test, or any other immunologic abnormality, (as seen by a test for LE cells, a simple, visual way of recognizing their presence).

For SLE patients with symptoms of mild arthritis, taking aspirin may be all they need. Antimalarial drugs are suggested if aspirin and bedrest do not control the active stage of SLE or the typical rash of lupus. Only if aspirin and antimalarial drugs fail or if the SLE patient becomes critically ill, has emotional outbursts, and kidney prob-

202 THE TRUTH ABOUT ARTHRITIS CARE

lems should steroids be begun. However, if the first lupus attack is severe, then steroids are used at once.

The SLE patient is usually well advised to stay out of the sun. Exposure may produce a worsening of the disease or bring out the skin rash even if the patient has not previously been sensitive to the sun.

As in other rheumatic diseases, there are a number of drugs that may be used in succession. If steroids do not work, then nitrogen mustard, an anti-cancer drug, may be tried. Recently, an immunosuppressive agent, like the ones used in heart transplant patients, has been tried on a number of SLE patients by Drs. Carl M. Pearson and Eugene V. Barnett at U.C.L.A. School of Medicine. This is azathioprine (Imuran), which has been tried by itself or in combination with steroid drugs. Although the investigators are encouraged by their preliminary results, the use of azathioprine is still in its early stages, and considerably more testing and study will be needed before any patient who is not treated in a medical center will be put on this drug. But that this drug shows promise is of great interest, and it is part of an encouraging trend of testing new drugs for SLE so as to extend effective treatment.

Perhaps more encouraging is that a number of patients have done very well for a great many years using only the more generally available drugs. One of my patients, a nurse, has coped with her disease for about forty years. Recently, I treated her for what she thought was her twenty-eighth acute attack. It was severe, but she is well enough now to go back to work.

So do not become discouraged should a doctor diagnose lupus. It can be treated more successfully now than ever before, and can be controlled, often indefinitely.

What should alert you to a possible diagnosis of SLE?

The likelihood is good that you may first have a fever, perhaps even up to 105 degrees. You lose your appetite, lose weight, are weak, often profoundly so. You may develop anemia or a rash that typically covers the bridge of the nose and the cheeks in a butterfly-like shape. This is the characteristic butterfly rash of SLE; at its worst, it lasts, and the skin becomes scarred, pitted, and discolored so that patients supposedly look lupine, therefore the name lupus (wolf in Latin).

Almost all my patients have had joint complaints. Some have only pain, while others get swelling or limitations in the motion of their joints, often fleeting. Although the arthritis seen in lupus looks like rheumatoid arthritis, there is a major difference. There are no bone erosions. To determine this, you must have X-rays done.

In fact, diagnostic tests are very important in SLE. New ones are always being tried out. At the moment the key test is the one already discussed, for the presence of LE cells. The presence (in addition) of a false-positive syphilis test may also indicate SLE. As one might expect, there are a number of blood abnormalities in lupus patients. They develop antibodies to their own blood cells, whether white or red, and also against platelets, the particles needed for blood clotting; there is even an antibody against the nucleus of the white blood cell, the central globular mass within the cell.

The antibodies against the nucleus are known as "antinuclear" (no relation to atomic power). Their presence is especially significant in an early case of SLE, when only arthritis is present. If antinuclear antibodies are present, then you may possibly have the disease, but not necessarily so. They are also found in other diseases, in about a quarter of the rheumatoid arthritis patients, for instance. But when the antinuclear antibodies cannot be found, you definitely do not have SLE.

Finally, perhaps the most signal advance in lupus is the increasing interest shown in this disorder. Interest has brought wider knowledge, and this in turn has brought earlier, easier recognition. Inevitably, better diagnosis brings a greater focus on therapy. And all of this is reflected in the way lupus treatment is improving.

SCLERODERMA

It is as if the hardening of the arteries to which all aging humans are subject stiffens the body's largest organ, the skin. That is the way of scleroderma whose name derives from the Greek *skleros* (hard) and *derma* (skin). But as in so many other rheumatic disorders, the name is misleading. The disorder is more accurately described by the more all-inclusive term "progressive systemic sclerosis." It is a rare, relentless systemic disorder of connective tissue. The process of sclerosis primarily affects the elasticity of the skin, the joints, and, with often serious consequences, the kidneys, lungs, and heart.

Scleroderma most often plagues women, and most frequently begins when they are 40 or 50 years of age. The prospect of progressive sclerosis is quite frightening, especially since one cannot predict with any accuracy at all what the disease will have in store for a particular victim. Scleroderma may be rapidly fatal. More often, the disease follows a slow progressive course, with stops and starts, long periods of spontaneous remission are followed by sudden exacerbations. Death may be due to some complication or to an infection. The disease has been known to last 20 to 30 years, particularly if the systemic sclerosis is not severe.

Two early symptoms are characteristic tip-offs to the disease. Some patients for years before developing scleroderma suffer from Raynaud's phenomenon—hands and sometimes the feet become painful and turn blue when exposed to the cold.

The inability to swallow more than a small amount at one time is another frequent early sign. This is a dysphagia that may become quite troublesome. Cough or labored breathing after exertion are later symptoms that indicate that the lungs or heart are affected as part of the systemic sclerosis. A distinguished rheumatologist who specializes in this disorder, Dr. Gerald P. Rodnan of the University of Pittsburgh School of Medicine, demonstrated that while skin changes are often the first manifestations of scleroderma, changes in a number of internal organs may precede those of the skin by long periods of time, and on occasion, may cause serious illness long before the skin begins to harden.

However, the skin changes are most often seen and are perhaps the most upsetting aspect of the disease. The skin becomes thickened and hard, even leathery; this process begins in the arms and legs, and eventually spreads to the face and trunk. The body is encased, causing a "Roman breastplate" effect. When the face becomes extensively involved, it assumes a mask-like appearance. The skin is tightly drawn, all wrinkles and expression are lost. There is both a shininess and a tautness of the skin, a pinching of the nose, and even a certain puckering of the mouth. It is as if one's skin had become two sizes too small.

Aspirin helps with the arthritis complaints, while

steroids may make patients with lung disease more comfortable. Steroids may be harmful, however, when the kidney is already affected (unlike the situation in lupus where steroids are used to treat kidney complications). In such instances, steroids may cause great harm in the rapid increase of high blood pressure. This may perhaps even cause death.

The most useful measure in the early care of the scleroderma patient is a bit of coddling. They must wear gloves and warm footgear to prevent the painful symptoms of Raynaud's phenomenon.

Skin changes are accompanied by joint pain and some swelling. Rarely, however, does arthritis become severe as it does in rheumatoid arthritis.

There are various approaches that attempt to delay the hardening of the skin: physical therapy, the use of heat (not cold, because that will provoke Raynaud's phenomenon), followed by massage and gentle exercise. And there are drugs that aim to soften the skin or try to delay the hardening. About thirty have been proposed, but only a few are in use. Some of these are agents that remove accumulated calcium, or increase the supply of oxygen to the tissue. None of them are specific, or too successful.

No effective method for treating progressive systemic sclerosis is currently available. Rheumatologists and their patients "are still awaiting a really satisfactory treatment," according to Drs. John Lansbury and Rosaline R. Joseph of Temple University School of Medicine. "This will probably arise from a clearer understanding of the pathogenesis of the disease."

Scleroderma is clearly a disease whose study is just beginning. The first steps have been taken. This includes the understanding of the natural history and possible cause of scleroderma; the search is now on for drugs, old or new, that will prove effective, while all the time there is the determination to make a patient as comfortable as possible. These are the early signs that progress is being made, and that in the near future more progress may be expected; hopefully, much more progress.

WHEN ARTHRITIS PRECEDES CANCER

It is not too far-fetched to predict that the astute diagnosis of a form of arthritis may some day save your life.

This prediction may seem startling, but it is based on solidly documented facts that have been accumulated by rheumatologists who have become increasingly sophisticated in their understanding of arthritis and its possible and occasional link to cancer. The fact that the two occur simultaneously in the same person has been documented often enough to no longer make it seem unique or unusual.

Perhaps the most exciting of the many discoveries in the field of rheumatology, the link between arthritis and cancer, holds out a great deal of clinical promise. For it may be more than just another means of early cancer detection.

What makes the observation of the coexistence of arthritis and cancer so very interesting is that one appears to precede the other. In certain cancer patients, arthritis will be observed first, while cancer remains undetected, unobserved, and out of view, yet beginning its deadly growth. But if the arthritis is correctly interpreted—this is admittedly a big if—the hidden malignancy will be unmasked and removed quickly enough so that the life it threatens will at least be prolonged, if not preserved. For a few fortunate patients, this has already been a thrilling reality.

As you can see, rheumatology does run through other parts of medicine, as stated previously. The link between arthritis and cancer has a two-pronged importance. On the one hand is the clinical, the potential early detection of the cancer. On the other hand, there is the research promise, the solving of this mysterious puzzle posed by this seemingly unlikely coexistence.

Perhaps by understanding why this phenomenon occurs, more will be learned about *both* cancer and arthritis, and two of the most puzzling of the rheumatic disorders, systemic lupus erythematosus and dermatomyositis, the inflammatory disorder that affects the skin, the tissue beneath the skin, as well as the underlying muscle. Dr. Carl M. Pearson of U.C.L.A. School of Medicine and others have suggested that the coexistence of malignancy and rheumatic disease may be explained by the possibility that cancer cells cause an immunologic alteration that somehow triggers an arthritis or a connective tissue disorder. Unfortunately, far too often, the arthritis preceding or coexisting with cancer had not been properly or quickly enough recognized. Here are a few instances in which this phenomenon occurs:

• Clubbing or enlargement of fingertips and toes, enlargement of extremities, thickening of the scalp and skin, and arthritis may all be a sign of lung cancer. In fact, ten percent of lung malignancies are believed to be accompanied by this form of arthritis. Other possible cancers suggested by the clubbing are those that affect the thorax, the lining of the thoracic cavity, or the diaphragm. This form of arthritis is called secondary hypertrophic (the morbid enlargement or overgrowth) osteo-arthropathy (any disease of joints or bone).

The clubbing appears suddenly and is often accompanied by some pain in the fingertips or toes. And if the tumor is removed, the clubbing, which begins with thickening around the nail bed and a feeling of warmth and slight burning, just vanishes. It is really dramatic how quickly the appearance of fingers and toes returns to normal, and symptoms disappear. It is so swift that it may take just a few hours after the cancer operation, or perhaps days. But the arthritis disappears and so, hopefully, does the cancer. Clubbing that is not associated with cancer is painless; and happens very slowly, taking months or years.

• Secondary gout has often been linked to blood cancers such as polycythemia (too many red blood cells), leukemia, lymphoma, or multiple myeloma. Very high levels of uric acid and, sometimes, also gouty arthritis, are observed. It is the presence of severe kidney trouble when it accompanies secondary gout that will make a doctor suspect a cancer.

Suspicions about cancer are also aroused when a doctor sees a patient who is older than 50 who has just developed such secondary gout and who cannot remember anyone in the family ever having had the gout. Such a lack of family history together with the peculiar triad of findings should alert the doctors to a blood cancer, according to Dr. Ts'ai-fan Yü, who, with Dr. Alexander B. Gutman of New York's Mount Sinai School of Medicine, has done so much to improve care for the gout patient.

• Juvenile rheumatoid arthritis has preceded leukemia in four of my patients. It was the low hematocrit (measurement of volume of red blood cells compared to the whole blood volume) that determined the underlying disease. It took a good deal of time to come to the proper diagnosis, from 4 to 24 months in the children whose ages were 22 months and 5, 9, and 15 years respectively. But fortunately not too long. Each child could be helped. The disappearance of bone and joint pain was often one of the first indications that the treatment for leukemia was working.

There are a number of other, even rarer, arthritic conditions in which the suspicion of cancer should be considered for as long as it cannot be definitely disproved. Anemia, weakness, or bone pain in a patient above the age of 50 might suggest multiple myeloma. Malignant lymphoma has been associated with diseases like SLE, dermatomyositis, rheumatoid arthritis, and other rarer rheumatic conditions. But their specific names are not as important as the simple determination to get a thorough examination by a legitimate and knowledgeable practitioner. In the past, the fact that arthritis can signal cancer has been largely overlooked, because it was just not sufficiently known. This too has changed. It is but one of the many advances of modern rheumatology.

But I feel that this is only the beginning. In his book, *Systemic Lupus Erythematosus,* Dr. Edmund L. Dubois cites a beautiful quotation on change and improvement in the knowledge of diseases: "Take pneumonia. It has been treated by brandy, and got well. It has been left to itself, and got well. And the bleeders, the brandy givers, and the doers of nothing at all, respectively, have had a vast deal to say for themselves and against their rivals. And which of them are to be our guides and masters in the treatment of pneumonia? None of them for a single day, much less for always."

So it is with arthritis. There is slow but steady change and learning. There is hope and improvement. There is always change, since even the expert's opinion may last only for a single day, so that on the day following a better, more effective treatment may be started.

VIII. *The Fleeced Americans:*
What You Should Know About
Quacks and Frauds

The curse of man, and the cause of nearly all his woe, is
his stupendous capacity for believing the incredible.
                                                H. L. Mencken

It has been estimated that consumers waste $500 million
a year on medical quackery . . . Unnecessary deaths, in-
juries, and financial loss . . . can be expected to continue
until the law requires adequate testing for safety and
efficacy of products and devices before they are made
available to consumers.
                                                John F. Kennedy

FOR SOME TIME NOW I have been half expecting some
enterprising quack to advertise moon dust as an arthritis
cure. It is about the only thing left that the gullible have
not paid dearly for. When some rocks or dust brought
back by an Apollo crew disappeared, I felt sure that
moon dust would soon be available. But the stolen sam-
ples were recovered, and I felt relieved. Still, there remains considerable other "dust" recklessly tossed into the
eyes of the unwary arthritis victims, be it a copper bracelet, complicated, expensive, worthless machinery, expensive
sessions in a "radioactive" cave, or lengthy and ineffectual
treatment in a sanitarium that specializes in self-styled
"natural healing methods."

These are all ugly dodges to defraud the arthritis victim. They are dangerous because treatment is postponed while the disease advances, while also destroying the spirit of hope each patient must maintain in order to fight his disease.

I did not know when I started to treat arthritis patients that I would be in constant competition with quacks and quackery—and furthermore that I would be repeatedly in danger of losing my fight to provide proper treatment. But this is exactly what I have experienced time and time again.

Sometimes I wish I were as diverting or as vivid as some personable charlatan! And then I daydream that I will devise a remedy that is both medically sound and as simple and enthralling as the discredited vinegar and honey "cure" for arthritis. Or·that I will invent something as popular as the copper bracelet with its unproved but magic capacity to prevent arthritis. Except, of course, my invention would work!

Such fantasies are the result of the frequent and painful frustrations of my profession. There is truly no worse experience than to watch helplessly while a patient turns down treatment that would help in order to embrace some nonsense that will be the beginning of a long and painful self-destruction. Quackery is a cruel waste of money, opportunities, and sometimes even life. Perhaps it is fortunate then that some people who do not fully trust organized medicine also distrust the quack and his products. They want the best of both worlds, or at least they try.

Marvin F., charming and intelligent, an athlete, chess expert, and a songwriter, wears a mock gold and elephant hair "copper" bracelet. Incidentally, Marvin is surprisingly well-informed about medicine. But there is no really convincing him that the copper bracelet will not do a thing to prevent the recurrence of the "tennis elbow" that has bothered him repeatedly during the past few years. Actually, he now protects his elbow a little and does not put quite as much stress on it as once he did. That is probably why Marvin has had less trouble with it recently. But he attributes it all to a series of bracelets he has worn—hard to get and expensive, he points out, because they are in such demand. He insists the copper "works." But ask him how, and he becomes vague and mumbles something about "magnetic action on the blood . . . or that copper is one of the better conductors of heat, and that's always good for *any* arthritis, it also affects the acidity of the body, and, anyway, if copper bracelets have been around this long, there *must* be *something* to them." And I don't argue, because I am convinced that when and if Marvin's elbow ever bothers him again, he will assume the "magic" of his copper bracelet has failed to work, and will see his doctor for the proper care he needs. And that is what really counts.

Copper bracelets at least are decorative, and as far as I am concerned, it is all right for you to wear one, *if*—and it is a big if—you do not neglect your arthritis, if you do not depend on the bracelet alone.

I like what Dr. William E. Reynolds, the medical director of the Arthritis Foundation, has to say about "arthritis jewelry."

"Wearing a copper bracelet for relief of arthritis is comparable to wearing an amulet containing a dead toad to ward off evil spirits. One of the reasons this kind of superstitious remedy catches on is that arthritis may temporarily go away by itself. If this happens by coincidence when someone is wearing a copper bracelet, he is likely to think the bracelet did the trick."

Dr. Reynolds has also pointed out that metallic copper is not absorbed through the skin and, therefore, cannot exert an internal effect. Furthermore, some recent research suggests that rheumatoid arthritis patients, for instance, do not lack copper, but may be oversupplied, according to Dr. William Niedermeier of the University of Alabama. After analyzing and comparing normal and diseased joint fluid, he reported finding a three-fold greater concentration of copper in joint fluid he removed from a group of rheumatoid arthritis patients. The researcher also went on to demonstrate more copper in the blood of these patients, when compared to blood taken from some normal volunteers. Ironically then, it seems that in spite of the great copper bracelet fad, this metal is not what rheumatoid arthritis patients lack.

That copper from a bracelet cannot penetrate the body is a fact either unknown or ignored by people who wear these bracelets to prevent or improve a great variety of diverse muscle and bone conditions, and are willing to pay up to $100 for the dubious privilege.

A statement by the Arthritis Foundation puts things in their proper perspective:

"Copper bracelets can't do you any harm. If you like jewelry, and copper jewelry in particular, we recommend them—whether you have arthritis or not. If you have some kind of arthritis and a copper bracelet makes you feel better, great! But don't wear it *instead* of getting proper diagnosis and treatment. If you have a serious kind of arthritis which can get steadily worse, putting off proper treatment could mean unnecessary pain and even permanent crippling."

I don't like to dwell on or poke fun at the credulity of friends or arthritis patients, and for a number of reasons.

It is so *human* to believe, as do Marvin, golfer Bert Yancey, and literally hundreds of thousands of other people, that someone somewhere has discovered that a copper bracelet will ward off arthritis. In fact, just now the old copper bracelet fraud—considered by some quackery experts probably the oldest and perhaps most vicious arthritis swindle—is having quite a revival, discouragingly enough among the young, and especially among sports enthusiasts. They should know better. After all, they are children of this scientific age.

For the *now* approach to arthritis care, and to protect yourself against arthritis quackery, avoid the following hazards to your health and pocketbook:

• Avoid ill-advised, sometimes unscrupulous, doctors who dispense either ineffective drugs or those that are potentially dangerous. In Georgia, California, and Kentucky are doctors who inject vitamins. In Ohio, a doctor has advertised his medical treatment that consists of a whirlpool bath filled with various herbs and drugs. Two physicians in Florida have caused kidney damage to their patients by giving overdoses of gold salts. In Port Arthur, Texas, in Canada, and Mexico, doctors give Liefcort, the drug that did so much damage to Rachel Warner and other patients of mine.

If you have any doubts about your medical treatment, and you do not find the answer in these pages, please do yourself the favor of checking with the people who run your local Arthritis Foundation! Write them, if you are not close to a local chapter.

• Beware of devices that are sold through the mails, electrical instruments that use magnetic induction to "cure" arthritis, anything that is supposedly "radioactive" (fortunately, it never is), or uses plain old-fashioned electricity.

• Stay away from chiropractors, or osteopaths who have not been trained in one of the modern, enlightened osteopathic colleges, and *all* naturopaths.

• Be very cautious if you are tempted to try a faith healer. Belief in faith healing says something about your attitude about yourself and your disease—you are tempted to trust primitive healing rituals and folk healing. You are part of what psychiatrist E. Mansell Pattison has called contemporary America's "continuum of magical belief systems that range from witchcraft to Christian Science." You are repressing reality when you refuse to accept facts, such as the high incidence of deaths from cancer reported among Christian Scientists.

• Don't let yourself be swayed by the blandishments of so-called arthritis clinics that advertise in books, magazines, and through the mails. They promise you all manner of fabulous treatments, although most of them use "natural" methods—starvation diets, purgatives and enemas, and lying in the sunshine. Milk farms, health resorts, or spas can be fine for a rest, to get away from it all. But don't consider them for a minute as arthritis treatment centers, unless they also have arthritis specialists, legitimate ones, on their staff. Again, check with your local chapter of the Arthritis Foundation to see if a clinic is really a worthwhile rehabilitation center.

Perhaps you should write to Jerry Walsh and consult with him, as I have often done. Jerry is the consultant on quackery to the New York headquarters of the Arthritis Foundation and is also on the President's Committee on Employment of the Handicapped. He has not only studied how the vultures who prey on the gullible arthritis victims operate, he has done what others would like to do: he has entrapped a number of unprincipled healers and put them out of business.

Not too long ago, Jerry, with a microphone concealed on his person, consulted a notorious quack who was already under indictment. What was needed was additional evidence to put this man in jail. And the nonsense the bearded quack told Jerry about his disease did just that. For the microphone Jerry was carrying transmitted the conversation to a local TV and radio station.

Jerry, a man whom I greatly admire and whose friendship I value, is undoubtedly the country's leading authority on arthritis quacks and the duplicity they practice. He is also a man who has successfully coped with an extremely serious case of rheumatoid arthritis.

Since the age of 18, Jerry has been fighting a valiant battle against his rheumatoid arthritis. It caused him to be bedridden and to go through a period of relying on quack treatment. But while rheumatoid arthritis cut short Jerry's promising career as a professional baseball player, it has not stopped him. He is in there pitching. His zest for living is remarkable. Although he uses both a crutch and a cane, Jerry Walsh is the kind of man who will carry your luggage, and will not let you carry his.

Jerry may have had difficult moments during his dedicated sleuthing to help rid this country of those who take their profit from the misery of arthritis victims, but trying to educate the American public about arthritis has not been easy, either. Some time ago, Jerry appeared on a national TV program. On the show, he demonstrated a number of quack devices and then went on to explain and describe why they were worthless.

The response to his appearance was fantastic. Within a few days he received close to 5,000 letters. But most of

the people wrote in to ask Jerry where to obtain the use-
less devices, and he was overwhelmed with requests to
supply the names and addresses of the vultures whom he
had just denounced. Since Jerry's life is dedicated to understanding exploited arthritics and their all-too-under-
standable and human desire to find help, he refused to be
discouraged. A lesser man would have been crushed.

Jerry Walsh has collected close to 500 medicines and
gadgets, a few of which he carries with him in a "little
quack bag." On crutch and cane, he continues to travel
the country, visiting a hundred or more cities in one year
and covering 100,000 miles or more. He displays the
gadgets he has been offered—their original cost ranged
from $22.50 to $900, while their medical worth is absolutely zero—and keeps busy alerting doctors, arthritis patients, and anyone else who will listen to the dangers of
fake arthritis devices, clinics, "cures," and misprescribed
drugs.

It is to everyone's benefit to listen to and learn from
Jerry Walsh, the man with the message of truth for the
estimated 90 percent of American arthritics who at some
time have fallen victim to one or another form of quackery!

One of the widely quoted stories Jerry tells, and my
favorite, concerns a member of my profession, a respected
arthritis specialist, who carries a horse chestnut on his
person at all times, since chestnuts or buckeyes are
reputed to have magic curative powers.

"Reason tells me it won't help," this doctor has told
Jerry, "but—who knows?"

This is what Jerry and I are fighting all the time. It is
the struggle within oneself between belief and disbelief,
between reason and unreason. The doctor whom Jerry
quotes is not a quack; he provides the best arthritis care

he can. He is merely practicing the ancient and honorable art of denying reality. He is extremely human in that he refuses to face some hard-to-tolerate facts, because this is the easier way and because this is how you avoid anxiety. Denial is the ruse many of us cling to when we continue to go on smoking, all the while accepting the awful facts about cigarettes and their role in causing stomach ulcers, heart disease, and lung cancer. But we only hurt ourselves.

As I have stated before, it is so very *human* to be always looking for new treatments. We all do that. And of all those in search of new ways of relief, few have a more difficult time than patients with arthritis. Theirs is a familiar complaint: Many, after years spent in disappointing experiences with their diseases and their doctors, have concluded, often justly, that doctors know little or nothing. And when they meet, they talk and reinforce their conviction on this matter. I have heard my patients say just that in my waiting room. My diagnosis then is not just arthritis but also apathy, and I know I must do something about both conditions.

If a new drug or treatment does come along, either approved or denounced by arthritis experts, the brotherhood whose lodge is arthritis will hopefully embrace it. The word is out with incredible speed that this is it! Just the very existence of something new is cheering. And it is, sadly enough, so human that the more simple-minded and far-fetched the promise of whatever is new, the greater the hopes of the arthritis brotherhood. But then, when you are hurting, caution becomes meaningless. Blame the resulting lack of logic on the pain of the body that coexists with a hunger in the heart to be as once you were. Compromised judgment and dispensed disbelief, those great close friends of quackery, take over.

Quackery was born when the first villain met the first fool, stated Voltaire. But I agree only in part; quacks are *villains*, but you don't have to be foolish to be credulous or to want to believe the incredible. All it takes is for one to be human. It is so human to believe that there is someone much smarter than anyone else. For, if one believes, one has hope, and that is man's most attractive characteristic! But having to sustain hope also makes man vulnerable, none more so than the most fleeced Americans of them all, the arthritis victims. Quacks know this and act on the knowledge that "there is scarcely anyone who may not, like a trout, be taken by tickling." Unfortunately, that is the way it has always been.

There were great numbers of quacks in Roman times, and in every period of history since then. And all quacks throughout all time have had something simple in common—the way the product they pushed was sold. Emotional packaging, you might call it. No matter what the product was, and no matter when it was sold, it was made attractive by being outside the conventional medicine of the time.

That is the tickling today, exactly as it was two thousand years ago.

Inevitably, you, the public, are the loser. United States arthritis victims are vulnerable to the tune of $400 million a year. People who fall for fraudulence and quackery really believe that quackery is a thing of the past—that it went out with hootchy-kootch dancers, river boat gamblers, and snake oil peddlers. Of course, the opposite is true. The rogues who gull the poor and the polished charlatans who prey on the rich are doing better than ever! Only their style has changed. They have turned from tub-thumping to television commercials, to high-powered direct mail, and to glossy illustrated pseudomedical brochures. The techniques are shiny-new, but the approach is usually antique. It did not surprise me to read recently that a quack was put in jail because he sold some wonder cure he had gotten out of Nicholas Culpepper's *The English Physician*, a book that was considered of dubious medical merit in the 17th century.

Long ago I stopped scolding patients when they refused to face facts and indulged their wishful thinking through the use of quack devices. I had been seeing a great many patients who had been hideously and needlessly harmed by quacks and was seething with indignation about any suggestion of quackery. Then I examined the feet of a sweet, diffident, and elderly nun. Much to our mutual embarrassment, I discovered that she was wearing a thin copper circle around her ankle. She had obviously not expected me to examine her feet, and I found myself wondering what I should say. But then I took my cue from her gentle forbearance. I reassured the sister and told her it was all right to keep wearing the anklet, just as long as she promised me that she would faithfully follow my prescribed treatment. We were both made happy; the sister was relieved I did not insist that she take off the anklet, while I was pleased that she did as I asked.

Actually, most of my educational efforts are aimed at physicians. In 1964, when I testified before Congress, I expressed my fears about the harm that doctors can do by not fighting quackery more wholeheartedly.

"Many physicians," I testified, "are unaware of the vast scope of the quackery problem; others excuse their disinterest by saying these promoters do not harm the patient and they actually give them some sort of psychological boost.

"The aspect that disturbs me most is that while these

remedies may not physically harm the patient, they indirectly injure him by postponing adequate treatment and arousing false hopes. Repetitious disappointment of aroused hopes for obtainable relief brings discouragement to the patient and makes him suspicious of all treatment—even that which can legitimately help. It is not by accident that nearly 50 percent of those who believe they have rheumatism are not under medical supervision, and many of them are not under a doctor's care because they believe little can be done for them.

"Every physician owes it to his patient to become aware of this multimillion-dollar exploitation and to cooperate actively with those attempting the often difficult task of protecting the arthritis sufferer . . ."

Most often doctors are helpless in trying to stop a patient determined to turn to quack remedies. Often such people have only consulted a physician to convince themselves that nothing can be done for them by conventional medicine. They are among the surprising number of people who prefer to chance magic, faith or folk healers, soothsayers, or the dangers of mentalistic healing—the Christian-Science type that centers on the denial that disease exists. Call it magic, fundamentalist-pentecostal, the believers are devout and cannot be deterred. They may suffer and even perish, but they do not complain. Little, if anything, can be done about these patients and their firm disregard of the realities of their situation.

But it is similarly disappointing that in too many instances doctors are responsible for their patients turning to quack cures. They are, after all, only human, just like their patients.

The type of doctor who inspires his patient's distrust and suspicion is often technically trained, rather than truly educated in the human sense. This physician may rely almost exclusively on a large number of laboratory tests, maintains an inflexible, overbearing air of omniscience, is remote, impersonal, and even authoritarian. He actually drives a patient into the arms of a personable, interested quack.

Another type of doctor may have all the medical and human skills, but is unable to communicate with his patients. It is a pity that only recently has the medical profession taken an interest in the communication skills. For instance, a recent survey at London Hospital points up the importance of the doctor's ability to have his patient understand what he is told. At the 1970 British Medical Association scientific meeting, Dr. M. Mason reported that patients at the hospital's clinic remembered less than half what their doctors said, and some managed to remember exactly the opposite of what they had been told. Not a single patient remembered all ten items discussed at the visit under study, said Dr. Mason. Doctors, it was discovered, differed not only in the information they supplied about a disease, but also in their ability to make the facts stick. Dr. Mason suggested that the individual need for medical information should be diagnosed as carefully as the need for medication. Doctors, he pointed out, are often counseled to dispense reassurance, but it is of no value if it does not register.

And then, quite the opposite of misunderstanding and neglect, there is something mysterious that happens in medicine. It flows from the sincere interest of an optimistic doctor who can by the simplest efforts play an enormous role in helping a patient. This may be called "cure by love." It is not an illusion, neither is it quackery. I have known a few physicians who were healers in the truest sense. They are rare and treasured, and at best we, their students, can only try and emulate them. For these are unusual human beings as well as inspired doctors and teachers. I suspect that if there were more like them, there would probably be no need or room in this world for quacks or quackery.

IX. *Even Doctors Ask: How Good Is Available Arthritis Care?*

DOCTORS HAVE BEEN often and sometimes unjustly accused of a conspiracy of silence about the services they provide their patients. This is no longer true. At first questions about quality were asked softly and privately, but now they are in the open, and to stay. Evaluation of medical services and the delivery of health services is a hotly debated public issue.

For you as an arthritis patient, these discussions are only a beginning of a far-reaching revolution. You have long asked the same question posed by one of the great physicians of this century, the late Russell L. Cecil, a pioneer in the field of rheumatology. He was the first to ask publicly whether patients with rheumatoid arthritis were receiving "the best possible treatment." What he thought about this question appeared in *Arthritis and Rheumatism*, the journal of the American Rheumatism Association, in April 1958:

"The question would have to be answered in the negative. Anyone who has had the opportunity to follow these patients, either in the hospital clinic or in private practice, knows that in the majority of cases some sort of compromise must be made with the ideal therapeutic program. In this respect, the arthritic is less fortunate than the patient with heart disease—most cardiacs can be well treated in the home with a minimum of physical manipulation. The same is true of patients with tuberculosis and many other chronic ailments. Why, then, is it so difficult for the rheumatoid patient to get first-rate medical care? One reason is purely geographic. Probably more than half live in rural or suburban communities where there are no adequate facilities for physical therapy, particularly hydrotherapy . . . Another cause for compromise in treating the arthritic is the financial one. Most patients have limited incomes. . . . A third reason for inadequate care of the arthritic is the inexperience and indifference of many family physicians. . . ."

There have been many changes in the years since Dr. Cecil wrote those pessimistic words. But although there has been change and improvement, not enough has taken place. The answer to the question of whether today's arthritis patients are receiving first-class care must regrettably remain, *no, they are not.*

Fortunately, one aspect of arthritis care has changed. In 1958, Dr. Cecil put part of the blame of poor care on the inexperience and indifference of many family physicians. He urged medical schools and hospitals to see that their "young graduates in medicine are better oriented in the field of rheumatic disease than they have been in the past, and that in particular they give more thought and attention to the care of the rheumatoid patient." Much has been achieved in this endeavor.

This can be seen at the annual meeting of the American

Medical Association. The most crowded areas are those where patients and doctors cooperate in "live arthritis clinics." Each year more interest has been shown when the specialists discuss patients and treatment approaches.

The growth of doctor interest in arthritis can be seen in the growing number of physicians who belong to the American Rheumatism Association. Before 1950, there were perhaps two hundred or three hundred members. In 1958, when Dr. Cecil wrote his despairing judgment about the quality of care for rheumatoid patients, there were considerably fewer than a thousand; today there are more than twice this number.

However, rheumatology is still a relatively new subspecialty in medicine. Although more physicians are entering the field, there are still far from enough, and certainly far too few to meet the needs of all who have some form of arthritis.

Obviously, all patients with rheumatic disease cannot be cared for by specialists—be they rheumatologists (who most often are internists), pediatricians, or surgeons. There are just not enough to go around. Lack of numbers, however, should not rule out first-rate medical care. Experience has shown that all physicians can provide very effective care.

If the best treatment is not generally or easily available, this may be so because not enough general doctors have kept up with the most recent advances. I am aware of this because so many patients are sent to me who have been overtreated, given drugs that are too potent, or who have otherwise been somehow mishandled by their family doctors.

Increasingly, however, value judgments are being made. Slowly and surely the capacities of doctors are being tested. For instance, in 1969, Dr. Donald D. Weir of the University of North Carolina reported the results of a unique evaluation of how doctors treat rheumatoid arthritis patients. The study, done in a Southern state, included about two hundred doctors—118 general practitioners, 60 internists, and 20 surgeons (the latter two, the specialists who most often see arthritis patients). Dr. Weir's aim was to find out what, if any, difference existed between the care of these three types of doctors.

The study included asking the doctors questions as well as sitting-in while they treated their patients. And the result showed that the internists as a group were perhaps the most helpful to their patients.

Dr. Weir found that the internists spent more time with their arthritis patients, learned more about them, kept better records, and perhaps did more thorough diagnostic work as shown by more frequent laboratory tests. Most important, however, was the finding that internists kept in touch with their patients more consistently than either the general practitioners or the surgeons. But the orthopedic surgeons (who also were interviewed and observed in actual practice) did extremely thorough examinations. The surgeons undertook more frequent X-ray examinations and more often ordered laboratory analysis of fluid drawn from a diseased joint.

Another significant observation that Dr. Weir reported was that the quality of advice about exercise and physiotherapy, the physical management—really the cornerstone of arthritis care—related to the amount of time that a doctor spent with a patient. As you will learn in the next chapter, amount of time is a crucial factor in evaluating the quality of care provided to an arthritis patient.

Dr. Weir's study also found that only eight of 198 physicians referred rheumatoid arthritis patients to a medical center where the most advanced and comprehensive treatment is usually available, since a so-called multidisciplinary team (rheumatologist, surgeon, physical therapist, psychiatrist, social worker, etc.) will attack all phases of a patient's problem.

This observation rather surprised me, and it bears out the judgment that quality arthritis care is too rarely provided to those patients who may need it. If I am surprised by what doctors do, what about patients? What recourse do they have?

What can a patient do who does not have access to the knowledge of a Dr. Weir and who cannot send a doctor as an advance man to determine how good another doctor is or how good the quality of the care is likely to be? That may be simpler than you imagined. You *can* judge your doctor's care, and fairly easily.

X. *How to Judge Your Doctor's Care*

WHEN YOU SAY you like your doctor that really means more than that yours is a good personal relationship. You may be surprised, but somewhere along the line you have judged your doctor's ability by a few simple things he says or does in the office. The idea of being both judge and jury of a doctor may seem alien to you. It occurs to me only because of the many articles I keep seeing that offer practical advice on how doctors can avoid being sued. Here are some of the rules proposed by several attorneys who specialize in medical liability cases:

• Never guarantee a cure. Be careful with your language. Don't say to a patient, "I'll make you as good as new" or, "You'll be as well as you were before." If a doctor makes such promises, the attorneys warn, he can be sued not only for negligence, but for breach of contract as well, if the good result fails to materialize.

• Keep up with advances in medicine. You will be judged by what is good medicine at the time of your

231

treatment. But don't keep too far up. If you experiment, announce it frankly as an experiment and get a written, informed agreement for the procedure. Unless there is a therapeutic reason not to tell the patient, make a simple, full, and complete disclosure of the risks involved. If the patient cannot be told for some reason, tell the patient's relatives. But get an informed consent for what you do.

• Keep good records. Records are witnesses who never die.

• Don't be hesitant about consultation. The greatest protection before juries is evidence that consultations took place.

• Maintain good public relations. Juries are influenced by the fact that doctors often refuse to make house calls and are sometimes offhand with their patients.

SEVEN SIMPLE SUGGESTIONS

It is interesting that the seven guidelines I suggest you use for deciding whether your doctor is doing the best in line with current standards are very little different from those the attorneys propose to keep doctors from being called to account in front of judge and jury. But then that only means that you should be aware that in the doctor-patient relationship what is good for one is also always good for the other. You are in this together. Therefore, you should know the following:

1. Right from the start, your doctor should not be vague. That is one of the most important elements of good care. Almost always, your doctor will arrive at an exact diagnosis and will then explain how he made his decision, what the main points of therapy will be, and what you may expect from treatment. If he cannot give you a clear-cut diagnosis, he will explain why he can't

explain—what baffles him about your case. He may at once suggest the option of consulting a specialist or a large medical center, or why you should trust him until a consultation is necessary.

2. A good doctor will invest time in a patient, especially at the beginning, when he must educate you about your disease. Do not expect an all-day "teach-in." But you should expect sufficient attention so that you are not vague about what you have. You should walk out of the doctor's office after a visit or two knowing clearly what your problem is, and if he cannot tell you this soon, you should know why this is so. You should have the doctor's assurance that he has time for you now and through the months and years when you make return visits.

3. A good physician will not promise you a cure, unless, of course, he is treating you for acute and self-limiting conditions, such as a bursitis or tendinitis.

When a physician assures you that he has never met a patient he could not help, he makes sense. But beware when he says that he will cure you of your rheumatoid arthritis or osteoarthritis, or that he will cure your child's juvenile rheumatoid arthritis, your son's ankylosing spondylitis, or your gout. You are in trouble. Perhaps you misunderstood the physician. Ask him to explain. If you do not have one of the self-limiting, acute rheumatic conditions, but indeed one of the rheumatoid diseases, you will know from the "promise of cure" that the doctor is not equipped either medically or emotionally to care for a serious and difficult long-term chronic condition. Furthermore, the "I'm gonna cure you" approach is frequently the sign of the quack or the self-appointed faith healer.

There is danger also that when a patient is promised a cure he will neglect himself. Most patients with rheuma-

toid arthritis experience relief or remission of their symptoms during the second year of disease. That may be a
mixed blessing, because this is the time when many arthritis patients tend to stop seeing their doctors. Those
who have been promised a "cure" are most cruelly deceived, for the disease is certain to recur. When it does,
they will feel cheated and hopeless as well.

In the treatment of rheumatoid arthritis, you have
really no way out. You must take the long view. You
should think of the third, fourth, or fifth year of disease
whether the disease is active or not. And tell yourself that
treatment during the disease-free year may prevent later
flare-ups.

4. A good physician does not rely on drugs only. If the
visits to your physician consist of exchanging notes on a
drug, if you are being given two or three drugs to take at
the same time, and drugs are changed frequently, then
you should seek medical attention elsewhere.

Drugs are, to my mind, the least important part of the
"total care" of your arthritis. Drugs are helpful, but remember they do not cure you. Drugs suppress inflammation, but as far as anyone can tell, they do not change
underlying disease processes. Therefore, it is what else a
physician does that matters.

Hallmarks of good therapy are evident in the time a
doctor takes to focus on preserving the function of an
affected hand or knee joint, and the exercises he prescribes and demonstrates to maintain such function and
to prevent joints from becoming "restricted" from disuse.

The arthritis specialist often sees patients who have
been through all the available drugs within the first year
or two of active disease. Some doctors prescribe drugs
carelessly, even recklessly on occasion, hoping they will
work. But that is the short-range approach. As I have said

before, if you have a chronic condition, you must take a long-range view; your care must provide physical as well as psychological comfort. The manner in which that is accomplished demonstrates whether your doctor provides exemplary or mediocre medical care.

5. Does your doctor make you feel secure? Does he know you as a person, not just a patient? Is he being frank with you, or is he holding something back? Is he optimistic, reassuring? Does he do a lot of little things for you?

The average patient with chronic rheumatic disorder always has a dark cloud hovering overhead. Will he suddenly be much worse? Will he be crippled, bedridden, totally disabled? Some patients fear they will die from their disease. Occasionally I have found that these generally unfounded fears exist even when a patient is doing well. The patient dreads the day when his condition will suddenly be so bad that he will become inactive, will be unable to work or take care of the family. Such feelings can have an overwhelming impact—not just on the outlook of a patient but also on his disease. Depression, anxiety and fears, and other stresses—poverty, grief, family troubles, job problems, sexual conflicts—all are factors that can induce a flare-up of disease.

In these circumstances, the physician should be saying all along that he is able to help, that he will be right there if the patient does have a flare-up. If your doctor echoes your helpless feelings, it is time for you to change to another, more optimistic physician. You need someone who will be completely frank with you, yet certain he can be of help, so that, even if you must put up with some limitations, you can lead a productive life.

6. How does your doctor handle your request for a verification of his diagnosis? How does he respond to

your wish to be seen by an arthritis specialist or at a well-known clinic? These questions may arise early or later in the course of your disease. But no matter when you ask for a second opinion, a good physician will encourage his patient in this desire for another doctor's diagnosis. A good physician is never afraid to get additional help from consultation or referral to another (perhaps not always better qualified) physician. A knowledgeable physician will use the consultation constructively, as a means of checking his treatment program. Often, the assurance of an expert, in some cases a renowned physician, that everything possible is being done will do wonders for a patient's progress. It also helps cement a better relationship between you and your doctor.

A good physician will keep his patients informed about their disease (and some possibly new approaches) by as many means as possible—such as authoritative books or pamphlets available from the Government, a medical society, or the Arthritis Foundation.

7. Perhaps the simplest way of finding out how well qualified by temperament and training your physician is to deal with a rheumatoid disease is your own reaction to him. Do you relate to him as a human being who has an interest in you? Is he on your side? Is he giving of himself?

Not all physicians are necessarily suited to the patients they treat—that is one of the reasons that specialization is so popular. Not all doctors can treat patients with chronic diseases; you make a common mistake when you assume that they can.

Remember that every doctor is a human being like you. His capabilities and interests vary, just like yours.

If you don't care for your doctor, change him; get yourself someone else. There are several ways of doing it.

Your county medical society can be of help. The offices of the local chapters of the Arthritis Foundation usually can provide the names of specialists and may also list a local arthritis clinic.

If your current medical treatment consists of a "paper exchange"—that is, the doctor gives you prescriptions for drugs and you hand over your money and that is all that's happening—forget it. Your dissatisfaction is normal. And don't be concerned if you have to see two or three or even four doctors before you feel happy with the physician.

If you do not want to go through so much self-questioning, merely answer this group of questions:

Do you like and trust your doctor? Does he like you? When was the last time you had a heart-to-heart talk?

Does he take enough time with you? Can you list the laboratory tests he does routinely? And why they are being done?

Have you ever discussed consulting another doctor who specializes in your problem? What was your doctor's reaction?

What drugs are you taking? Do you understand why you are taking these drugs? How often in the past year has your prescription been changed? Why was this change necessary?

Should you not be able to answer all these questions, either in the affirmative or by clear-cut explanations, then you should consider another physician.

SHOP FOR A DOCTOR, BUT DON'T BECOME A "DOCTOR-SHOPPER"

There is a great difference between a patient who sensibly "shops around" for a physician and the professional "doctor-shopper."

This latter arthritis sufferer is usually poorly motivated and looks for instant relief and "magic wands" to be waved. Most often this is a woman who has not come to terms with herself or with the nature of the disease.

The doctor-shopper often has heard of the country's top arthritis experts, and may have consulted all of them, but has accepted none of their advice. It is not uncommon for a rheumatologist to discover, after some questioning, that he is the eighteenth physician the patient has consulted. Doctors find such patients depressing and time-consuming, for very few can achieve sufficient insight to realize they are denying the facts of their disease. If the eighteenth physician advises the same things as the previous seventeen, and none of the advice has been taken, there is little left to do except refuse to treat the patient.

Occasionally, a physician will try to point out that such patients are unrealistic in seeking immediate relief, that they will never find a drug that will "cure," that they must content themselves with taking aspirin four or five times daily and exercising regularly and methodically.

Rarely can a physician break through the ironclad defenses of the confirmed doctor-shopper. They are pitiful, and their medical future is bleak since they face the torment of repeated disappointments. Invariably, these are the quack-prone patients who fall into the hands of the disreputable (sometimes even a doctor). They travel far and wide on the spurious trail of "the" cure, which like the elusive bluebird of happiness may well be available right at home in the guise of sensible arthritis care.

I estimate that during the past 15 years, I have been involved in the long-term treatment of about 3,000 patients and have had some sort of contact with approximately 10,000 arthritis patients. Of the 3,000 patients whom I saw in a large medical center and who were treated by a team of doctors, nurses, and social workers, I think there were some 450 doctor-shoppers. Only 150 of them could be persuaded to change their ways, to buckle down to a realistic appraisal of what could be done for them.

Doctor-shoppers come and go so quickly that too often they are not recognized for what they are. For those who could be helped, I found it useful to involve husbands, wives, fiancés, or other members of the family. All were asked to read arthritis literature, and the medical center's social workers helped to convince them that their first need was to stop doctor-shopping. They do not readily admit having consulted all those other doctors or that they know and may rely on various quack devices.

The lady who "doctor-shops" can be easily spotted by her dependence on neighborhood "curbstone advice" for the care and cure of arthritis. She always listens to the opinion she has just received. While she willingly accepts the neighbors' suggestions, or the far-out claims she may read in a magazine article, she is reluctant to listen to a qualified physician. Her attention span is short. She never maintains a complete regimen for the care of her arthritis, and she loses finally, since she is the kind of patient who postpones proper diagnosis and treatment until it is really too late to do too much for her. And then, of course, she puts the blame on doctors who can't do a thing for her.

XI. *Do You, Patient, Take This Doctor?*

IN THIS FINAL CHAPTER, I am going to surprise you by not discussing all the new drugs and new approaches that will radically change the future for arthritis patients. Instead, I am going to talk about you! And your relationship to your doctor—even give some advice on how you can improve your working together.

The promise for arthritis care exists and will be fulfilled, and in due time will be yours. We are forging ahead faster now than ever before. But the rapturous future is not what you are going to be offered right now. For instance, I know of at least 30 drugs that are currently being tested. But no one knows how good they are or when they will be generally available. Like yourself, I have also been reading more and more about the great strides that surgery is achieving, most recently by the use of new materials—jet age plastic and cement that may well be the answer to artificial "replacement" joints. New joints may even be transplanted. Undoubtedly, these advances will radically alter arthritis care in the future. But

what about the most difficult of all problems right now—
the *meantime,* the waiting until you can benefit from
what is new in the field?

The waiting game is the worst of trials. But there is an
advance that lies within yourself, there are strides you
can make today, and you need no one but yourself.

For if you want to get well, or can be stimulated to
want this, you will achieve remarkable results! This will
not get doctors off the hook, but it will make their responsibility to you far easier. That is what I have learned from
what I like to call the patient-physician "fit."

The way you relate to your doctor and he to you is the
key. You may compare it to a marriage. Some are good
fits, some are not.

It may seem almost as hard, however, to find a new and
good partner in long-term treatment as it may be to break
up a marriage that no longer fulfills your needs. But to
contract a new relationship that does work may well be
worthwhile.

This was borne home while I was in training at Harvard with Dr. Walter Bauer. This great rheumatologist
and teacher had been treating a rich, older lady with
rheumatoid arthritis. She had been coming to him for five
years, and despite everything he did, her condition gradually seemed to grow worse. She belonged to that tiny
percentage of patients with this disease for whom very
little can be done medically, in contrast to the 95 percent
of rheumatoid patients for whom a great deal can be
achieved.

It was surprising that this woman kept coming back,
satisfied with her treatment. And it amazed us that it was
Dr. Bauer, not she, who was in despair.

"Why are you coming back to me when we both know I
am not helping you?" he asked her. "Your disease is stead-

ily progressing downhill, and your physical limitations are becoming more apparent." For once a patient reas- sured a physician, for she insisted that he was helping her.

To Dr. Bauer's students it was apparent that he and this patient had created a kind of relationship that was meaningful and helpful. The patient could live with her disability and crippling because her physician had given something of himself that ranged far beyond his excep- tional professional competence. It was the deeply felt concern of one human being for another. The woman, in turn, was extremely receptive to his feelings of concern for her. And that was enough to help and sustain her.

It was Dr. Bauer who repeatedly asked himself, "What does this patient want from me?"

From him I learned that all doctors should ask them- selves the same question. Physicians need to recognize that very often patients expect more of them than they are able to give. Patients should be asked why they come back. Sometimes a great deal is revealed by the answer.

But you, the patient, should ask yourself the same question. Very often you do not realize that you should know why you are returning to the same physician, and what you expect in the way of help. Ask this question. You may find that a patient-physician "fit" is better than you had suspected.

In the body of this book I have repeatedly discussed the problem of arthritis care from both the doctor's and the patient's viewpoint. There still remain far too many problems, both medical and personal. But perhaps the leading difficulty for doctors is that far too many patients are spectacularly lax and ill-informed about their arthri- tis. If they knew as little about their jobs or keeping house, they could not function.

Unfortunately, just as the race is to the swift, so good medical care today is to the aware. The day of innocence in medical matters is past. The know-nothing patient is a poorly motivated patient. Full disclosure is the order of the day, and the care of chronic disease is more than ever a self-help, do-it-yourself project. Today, and specifically in arthritis, the doctor works *with* his patient, and the patient's responsibilities and duties are on a par with the physician's.

Almost invariably, arthritis and particularly rheumatoid disease is for life; it is difficult and capricious. Coping with it is easier for the initiated, knowledgeable patient. To do well a "good" patient must be both passionately and dispassionately involved—on the one hand, committed to his own interest; on the other, taking an informed, intelligent, well-motivated long view. But this is not easy to achieve. If it happens at all, it happens slowly.

Interestingly enough, the best patient is the kind of person who refuses to play "arthritis patient." These patients remain what they have always been; they refuse to label themselves "patients" or refuse to retreat helplessly behind the mask of being "hopeless."

Please remember that acute symptoms, no matter how severe, do not turn you from businessman or housewife into "rheumatoid patient." By having arthritis, a disease most often thought to relate to aging, you are not suddenly "over the hill" or finished with life. People with arthritis are not a species apart. You are just what you always were. And if you have some sort of trouble, this is the time to work on your difficulty. Become more self-reliant, not less so. Continue your life and improve on the quality of it; make accommodations to being sick only when and to the extent it is absolutely necessary.

Self-reliance, as much as what you do to cooperate with treatment, is the key to being an ideal arthritis patient. For many the help must come from within. Why not rely on yourself? Why not develop self-sufficience? One way of doing so requires little effort, no extensive probing into your past or present. It is simply a matter of knowing about yourself and your disease.

To a certain extent, you can doctor your own difficulties. See what you can learn from answering the following questions, which have been culled from an arthritis information survey prepared by Dr. Margaret H. Edwards for use at one of my clinics.

See how you answer to these questions. Most often a check mark is enough. Yet, you may be surprised by what you will learn about yourself—how much you already know or how little, or what you must still learn about yourself and your disease.

1. How long have you had arthritis?

   Less than 5 years _____
   Five to 10 years _____
   Over 10 years _____
   Don't know _____

2. What kind of arthritis do you have?

   Muscular rheumatism _____
   Bursitis _____
   Gout _____
   Lumbago _____
   Rheumatoid arthritis _____
   Lupus erythematosus _____
   Degenerative arthritis _____
   Spondylitis _____

Osteoarthritis ————————————————
Don't know ————————————————

3. What do you think caused your arthritis?

Hard work ————————————————
Inflammation ————————————————
Getting old ————————————————
Accident, injury ————————————————
Runs in family ————————————————
Blood too acid ————————————————
"Wear and tear" ————————————————
Dropped stomach ————————————————
Poor diet ————————————————
Bad teeth ————————————————
Climate, weather ————————————————
Nerves ————————————————
Dampness ————————————————
Weak constitution ————————————————
Altered chemistry ————————————————
Overweight ————————————————
Infection ————————————————
Bad blood ————————————————
Bad tonsils ————————————————
Other ————————————————
Don't know ————————————————
Nobody knows ————————————————

4. Where did you get the notion of what caused your arthritis?

Told by a doctor ————————————————
Told by a nurse ————————————————
Told by a relative ————————————————
Told by a friend ————————————————

Heard it said _____

Read it in newspaper, magazine _____

Read it in this book _____

Learned it from advertisement _____

Figured it out _____

Don't know _____

Have you now gotten the idea of how this questionnaire works? You should have precise answers to questions 1 and 2. But if you check degenerative arthritis, you
had better also check osteoarthritis, since they are the
same thing, and are the most frequently encountered
forms of arthritis. Question 3 is already more tricky. You
should really have answered only "Don't know" and "Nobody knows," and the more other factors you have
checked off, the more likely you are to be confused about
arthritis and mistaken in thinking something that you
have done has caused your arthritis. The same goes for
question 4. Your best source of what caused your arthritis
is the doctor and nurse and, hopefully, this book.

5. Do you think arthritis is curable?

Yes _____

No _____

Don't know _____

6. What medicine are you taking for your arthritis?

Alfalfa seeds _____

Anacin _____

Antimalarials _____

Aspirin _____

Benemid _____

Bufferin _____

Butazolidin _____

Cod liver oil _____

Colchicine _____

Cortisone _____

Darvon _____

Gold salts _____

Hormones _____

Liniments _____

New research or drug _____

Vitamins _____

Not listed _____

Don't know _____

7. What other forms of treatment are you presently taking?

X-ray _____

Exercises _____

Heat _____

Water treatment _____

Massage _____

Paraffin treatment _____

Lamp treatment _____

Salves _____

Electricity _____

Injections _____

Diet _____

Rest _____

Surgery _____

Osteopathic _____

Vinegar and honey _____

Stretching _____

Special apparatus (braces, tables,

exercisers, etc.) _____

Chiropractic _____

Other _____

Nothing _____

8. Do you believe aspirin affects the heart?

Yes _____

No _____

Don't know _____

9. Which of the above is, in your opinion, the best drug or treatment for arthritis? _____

10. Do you think you should be told more about your arthritis than you now know?

Yes _____

No _____

Don't know _____

11. Have you ever followed the advice of friends, relatives, or neighbors regarding how to treat your arthritis?

Yes _____

No _____

Don't recall _____

12. What advice have they given you?

Recommended a certain doctor _____

Recommended a certain medicine,
ointment, liniment, etc. _____

Recommended treatment by a private
person (healer, masseuse, etc.) _____

Recommended traveling or moving to
another climate _____

Recommended a certain clinic or hospital _____
Recommended a mineral springs or spa
for baths, packs, etc. _____
Recommended a special diet, certain foods _____
Recommended certain exercises,
manipulations, activities _____
Recommended religious practices,
relying on faith _____
Recommended other measures _____

13. Have you ever felt that a doctor who was treating you wasn't really interested in your arthritis?

    Yes _____
    No _____
    Don't recall _____

14. Have you ever thought that the treatments for arthritis were more troublesome or painful than the arthritis itself?

    Yes _____
    No _____
    Don't know _____

15. Do you believe your arthritis has made you an unattractive person?

    Yes _____
    No _____
    Don't know _____

16. Do you think your arthritis has affected your home life, or family life, in any way?

    Yes _____

No _____

Don't know _____

17. Do you think other persons have changed their attitude toward you since you have had arthritis?

Yes _____

No _____

Don't know _____

Question 5 may perhaps trip you up. Only self-limiting forms of arthritis are curable. Only if you have an acute infectious arthritis, or bursitis, can you clearly state that your arthritis is "curable." The list of medications in question 6 is incomplete, and you may not find what you are taking on this list. But if you check many medications, you are not being treated properly. You are obviously in trouble if you only take vitamins or cod liver oil.

In question 7, you should be checking the treatment approaches that are suitable to your specific form of arthritis, but not electricity, vinegar and honey, chiropractic, or nothing. If you answer question 8 in the affirmative, you are ill informed. If in question 9 you do not list the treatment you are now receiving, this may be a sign that you are dissatisfied with your present kind of care. The same is true if you answer yes to question 10. You should beware of being gullible if you answer 11 in the affirmative or more than the first and fifth parts in question 12. If you have answered questions 13 and 14 with a "yes," then you are really dissatisfied with your doctor, and should seriously consider seeking help from some other physician.

Should you have answered yes to questions 15, 16, and 17, you should discuss these feelings you have about yourself and your surroundings with your doctor. If he does not have specific suggestions for you, or has no time to discuss them with you, this may be a sign that you need another doctor or perhaps that you should have psychological counseling. But, in any case, you should air these feelings and not keep them to yourself.

Finally, answer this last question: In what way does your arthritis bother you?

Pain _____
Stiffness _____
Swelling _____
Fluid _____
Fever _____
Rash _____
Lumps, nodules _____
Joints deformed _____
       stiff _____
       not moving properly _____
       give way _____
Tired _____
Get discouraged _____
Nothing bothers me _____
Other _____

Make a copy of this list (and whatever you have checked off) and make a point to discuss your complaints with your doctor. You might be telling him something that you have not mentioned before. In fact, this whole questionnaire might serve as a basis for discussion about what is bothering you, as well as to tell you whether you know enough about your disease, and whether you have accepted the fact that you must learn to cope with your problem.

You should never lose sight of the fact that whatever your problem may be, you always have a valuable ally, your doctor. Use him well, and help him help you. How good a patient you are is crucial in determining what you will achieve in the doctor-patient relationship. Therefore, do you, patient, take this doctor? And will you bring to him your knowledge, your effort, and your confidence so that both of you together can conquer whatever afflicts you?

Not too long ago an advertisement for *Modern Medicine* delineated the remarkable relationship that exists between a patient and doctor. "There is no relationship like it in all the world," the advertisement stated, and I cannot help but agree. "It places a special responsibility on all of us to select with great care a physician in whose presence we feel comfortable and with whom we can freely communicate. And, perhaps, we should be willing to acknowledge, from time to time, that the person in whom we can place this trust and confidence is a rather special human being." But then, so are you. And there are no limits on what two special human beings can achieve by working together.

APPENDIX: *The Offices and Chapters of the Arthritis Foundation*

HEADQUARTERS AND EASTERN
AREA OFFICE
1212 Avenue of the Americas
New York, New York 10036
212—757-7600
Write to Headquarters if you
find no listing in your local
phone book.

ALABAMA
Alabama Chapter
13 Office Park Circle, Suite 22
Birmingham 35223
South Alabama Chapter
1367 Government Street
Mobile 36604

ARIZONA
Central Arizona Chapter
96 West Osborn, Suite D
Phoenix 85013

Southwest Chapter
3833 East Second Street
Tucson 85716

ARKANSAS
Arkansas Chapter
900 Marshall Street,
P.O. Box 125
Little Rock 72203

CALIFORNIA
Northeastern California
Chapter
1507 21st Street, Suite 300
Sacramento 95814
Northern California Chapter
166 Geary Street
San Francisco 94108
San Diego Area Chapter
3537 4th Avenue
San Diego 92103

Southern California Chapter
4311 Wilshire Boulevard
Los Angeles 90005

COLORADO
Rocky Mountain Chapter
1375 Delaware Street
Denver 80204

CONNECTICUT
Connecticut Chapter
964 Asylum Avenue
Hartford 06105

DELAWARE
Delaware Chapter
1900 Lovering Avenue
Wilmington 19806

DISTRICT OF COLUMBIA
Arthritis and Rheumatism
    Association of Metro-
    politan Washington
2424 Pennsylvania Avenue,
    Northwest, Room 112
Washington, D.C. 20037

FLORIDA
Florida Chapter
417 12th Street West
Perrine Plaza, Suite 3
Bradenton 33505

GEORGIA
Georgia Chapter
1038 West Peachtree Street,
    Northwest
Atlanta 30309

HAWAII
Hawaii Chapter
200 North Vineyard,
    Room 505
Honolulu 96817

IDAHO
Idaho Chapter
Eastman Building, Room 220
Boise 83702

ILLINOIS
Central Illinois Chapter
Allied Agencies Center
320 East Armstrong Avenue,
    Room 102
Peoria 61603

Illinois Chapter
159 North Dearborn Street,
    Room 515
Chicago 60601

INDIANA
Indiana Chapter
2102 East 52nd Street
Indianapolis 46205

St. Joseph County Chapter
521 West Colfax
South Bend 46601

IOWA
Iowa Chapter
914 Locust Street
Des Moines 50309

KANSAS
Kansas Chapter
240 Greenwood
Wichita 67211

KENTUCKY
Kentucky Chapter
1381 Bardstown Road
Louisville 40204

LOUISIANA
Louisiana Chapter
2801 Broadway
New Orleans 70125

MAINE
Maine Chapter
280 Front Street,
P.O. Box 333
Bath 04530

MARYLAND
Maryland Chapter
12 West 25th Street
Baltimore 21218

MASSACHUSETTS
Massachusetts Chapter
38 Chauncy Street, Room 611
Boston 02111

MICHIGAN
Michigan Chapter
27308 Southfield Road
Lathrup Village 48075

MINNESOTA
Minnesota Chapter
89 South 10th Street
Minneapolis 55403

MISSISSIPPI
Mississippi Chapter
104 Dale Building
2906 North State Street
Jackson 39216

MISSOURI
Eastern Missouri Chapter
Box 8100 1221 S. Grand Blvd.
Saint Louis 63156

Kansas City Chapter
2727 Main Street
Kansas City 64108

MONTANA
Midland Montana Chapter
1201 Avenue C
Billings 59102

North Montana Chapter
P.O. Box 2383
2095 2nd Avenue North
Great Falls 59401

Western Montana Chapter
1575 West Sussex Street
Missoula 59801

NEBRASKA
Nebraska Chapter
Southwest Plaza, Suite 306
4601 South 50th Street
Omaha 68117

NEW HAMPSHIRE
New Hampshire Chapter
Mail: Attn.
Mrs. Terry H. Van Brunt
P.O. Box 1010
Hanover 03755

NEW JERSEY
New Jersey Chapter
26 Prospect Street
Westfield 07090

NEW MEXICO
New Mexico Chapter
P.O. Box 8022
Albuquerque 87108

NEW YORK
Central New York Chapter
627 West Genesee Street
Syracuse 13204

Monroe County Chapter
973 East Avenue
Rochester 14607

New York Chapter
221 Park Avenue South
New York 10003

Northeastern New York
Chapter
11 North Pearl Street,
Room 602
Albany 12207

Western New York Chapter
220 Delaware Avenue
Buffalo 14202

NORTH CAROLINA
North Carolina Chapter
P.O. 2476
3100 Erwin Road
Durham 27705

NORTH DAKOTA
Dakota Chapter
325 South 7th Street
Fargo 58102

OHIO
Akron Area Chapter

326 Locust Street
Akron 44302
Central Ohio Chapter
1096 North High Street
Columbus 43201
Miami Valley Chapter
184 Salem Avenue
Dayton 45406
Northeastern Ohio Chapter
2239 East 55th Street
Cleveland 44103
Northwestern Ohio Chapter
3817 Monroe Street
Toledo 43606
Ohio Valley Chapter
2400 Reading Road
Cincinnati 45202

OKLAHOMA
Eastern Oklahoma Chapter
3815 South Harvard,
Room 13
Tulsa 74135
Oklahoma Chapter
825 Northeast 13th Street
Oklahoma City 73104

OREGON
Oregon Chapter
P.O. Box 42067
Portland 97242

PENNSYLVANIA
Central Pennsylvania
Chapter
P.O. Box 534
Harrisburg 17108

Eastern Pennsylvania
Chapter
311 South Juniper Street,
Suite 1008
Philadelphia 19107

Western Pennsylvania
Chapter
6115 Jenkins Arcade
Pittsburgh 15222

RHODE ISLAND
Rhode Island Chapter
49 Weybosset Street
Providence 02903

SOUTH CAROLINA
South Carolina Chapter
3202 Devine Street
Columbia 29205

SOUTH DAKOTA
Dakota Chapter (see North
Dakota)

TENNESSEE
Middle East Tennessee
Chapter
1719 West End Building,
West End Avenue
Nashville 37203

West Tennessee Chapter
2600 Poplar Avenue,
Suite 200
Memphis 38112

TEXAS
El Paso Chapter
Medical Arts Building,
Suite 304

415 East Yandell Street
El Paso 79902

Gulf Coast Chapter
4848 Guiton, No. 116
Houston 77027

North Texas Chapter
B-134 Blanton Tower
3300 West Mockingbird Lane
Dallas 75235

Northwest Texas Chapter
815 Eighth Avenue
Fort Worth 76104

South Central Texas Chapter
4322 Blanco Road, No. 3
San Antonio 78212

West Texas Chapter
2101 West Wall
Midland 79701

UTAH
Utah Chapter
1935 South Main, Room 635
Salt Lake City 84115

VERMONT
Vermont Chapter
215 College Street,
P.O. Box 422
Burlington 05401

VIRGINIA
419 North Boulevard
Richmond 23220

WASHINGTON
Inland Empire Chapter
604A Hyde Building
Spokane 99201

Western Washington Chapter
Seaboard Building, Room 526
4th and Pike
Seattle 98101

WEST VIRGINIA
4701 MacCorkle Avenue S.E.
Charleston 25304

WISCONSIN
225 East Michigan Street
Wisconsin Chapter
Milwaukee 53202

WYOMING
Rocky Mountain Chapter
(see Colorado)

Index

INDEX